LOOK, NOW HEAR THIS

LOOK, NOW HEAR THIS

Combined Auditory Training and Speechreading Instruction

By

JANET JEFFERS
Late Professor in Audiology
Department of Special Education
California State University
Los Angeles, California

and

MARGARET BARLEY
Instructor in Speechreading
Extended Campus Programs, Pasadena City College
Pasadena, California

Formerly, Professor in Speechreading
California State University
Los Angeles, California

With a Foreword by

Virginia McKinney
Director, Communicative Skills Program
for Multiply-Handicapped Adults
Los Angeles, California

CHARLES C THOMAS • PUBLISHER
Springfield • Illinois • U.S.A.

Published and Distributed Throughout the World by
CHARLES C THOMAS • PUBLISHER
BANNERSTONE HOUSE
301-327 East Lawrence Avenue, Springfield, Illinois U.S.A.

ISBN 0-398-03830-9
Library of Congress Catalog Card Number: 78-18503

With THOMAS BOOKS *careful attention is given to all details of manufacturing and design. It is the Publisher's desire to present books that are satisfactory as to their physical qualities and artistic possibilities and appropriate for their particular use.* THOMAS BOOKS *will be true to those laws of quality that assure a good name and good will.*

Printed in the United States of America
N-1

Library of Congress Cataloging in Publication Data

Jeffers, Janet.
Look, now hear this.

Includes index.
1. Deaf—Means of communication. 2. Lipreading. 3. Deaf—Education. I. Barley, Margaret, joint author. II. Title.
HV2487J42 362.4'2 78-18503
ISBN 0-398-03830-9

This book is lovingly dedicated to the memory of Doctor Janet Jeffers. She was an eminent contributor to the cause of the hearing-impaired and devoted her professional life to aid in their rehabilitation. Her academic superiority was nationally recognized. She was always modest and unpretentious about her outstanding accomplishments in the field of audiology. She leaves a noteworthy legacy to the profession.

M.B.

FOREWORD

Readers conversant with the scholarly presentation of the speechreading process detailed in their first book *Speechreading (Lipreading)* will find in this new text by Jeffers and Barley added dimensions to enrich the communicative rehabilitation process of hearing-impaired persons. The book is an outgrowth of the authors' many years of dedicated work in the area of aural rehabilitation, and it focuses on the presentation of pertinent theory and detailed procedures essential for successful simultaneous training in speechreading and auding in order to maximize overall communicative efficiency.

While the book presents only a brief overview of the auditory training process due to the untimely death of Doctor Janet Jeffers, this discussion is supplemented by the appendix which provides the professional reader with the definitive data about the auditory perception of phonemes used in the preparation of the auditory training materials.

Teachers and clinicians of speechreading will welcome the availability of the many new, diversified and creative materials presented in this volume. Clearly defined lesson format will serve as a model for development of supplemental materials using the technical data available in the appendix.

Virginia McKinney

PREFACE

IN ORDER TO HELP the hearing-impaired improve their communicative skill (understanding others and being understood by them) we professionals offer instruction under the general rubric of aural rehabilitation. Included are such activities as counseling, speech and language development or improvement, auditory training, and speechreading. This book is concerned with the two latter activities. Attentive listening and speechreading are two distinct but interrelated skills. The first skill, attentive listening (achieved through auditory training), consists of obtaining the maximum amount of auditory information from a defective receptive system. The second, speechreading, consists of using one's vision to complement what is received auditorily. Instruction in both skills, especially from a theoretical point of view, is markedly similar. Both include exercises designed to heighten sensory awareness, to ensure that important sensory information is not missed or ignored and is used in reaching perceptual closures, i.e. which phoneme?, which word?—often called "ear training and eye training." Both make use of similar materials—exercises and activities designed to improve one's associational skills in order to effect closure despite the fact that important auditory and/or visual information may be lacking. This kind of training (and eventual skill) is predicated upon one's knowledge of the language (contextual cues) and relies as well on situational and anticipatory cues (what one expects might be said or is frequently said in a given situation).

Stated differently, the most important and distinguishing feature between the hard-of-hearing and the deaf is the former's ability to hear accurately the vowels and diphthongs, the semivowels and the nasals (or at least nasal energy), and the aspirate. This is usually enough sound energy to enable him to develop normal voice quality and, with the aid of vision, linguistic competency as well. If the hard-of-hearing individual with a mild to moderate loss does not have normal voice quality even though his hearing aid(s) are adequate for his needs, it is possible that there is a central problem in auditory processing.

The aided audiogram can serve as a rough guide to the phonemes the client can be expected to recognize following training. To make this judgment one compares the frequency range of the phoneme in question with the frequency range of the audiogram. This will usually prove to be a very conservative judgment inasmuch as there are multiple cues to the recognition of consonant sounds. Some of these are the intensity of the voiceless energy which will be greater for the voiceless phonemes. The nature of the voiceless energy burst or a continuant helps to differentiate plosives from fricatives.

INTRODUCTION

DIAGNOSTIC HEARING TESTING PRIOR TO AUDITORY TRAINING

Relevance to Planning the Auditory Training Program

AUDITORY TRAINING in the United States has for the most part been limited to teaching children gross discrimination tasks (bell, horn, drum) and adults finer discrimination (fin, thin, sin). In many instances it has been *highly unsuccessful* because the child's or adult's ability to hear has not been considered. Sound makers of high frequency and low intensity, e.g. crickets, have been presented to children whose residual hearing was below 1000 Hz. Often no attempt has been made to insure association of sound with important nonlinguistic events, e.g. vacuum cleaner, garbage disposal, water running, toilet flushing, etc. The adult has been asked to differentiate among /f/, /θ/, and /s/ (fin, thin, sin) when a glance at his aided audiogram, i.e. threshold levels when wearing hearing aid, would have made patently clear that such a task would be impossible.

The habilitative audiologist setting goals and selecting materials for his hard-of-hearing clients should be guided by up-to-date pure tone and speech audiometry results. The latter serves as a guide to what phonemes the pupil can now recognize with amplification; the former serves as a guide to speech sounds not now recognized that should be recognized following adequate training.

No one should be expected to recognize phonemes on the basis of limited information when full information is available with a better amplifier. Before initiating auditory training one needs to be assured that the client's hearing aids are providing him with maximum help—that he is hearing as well with them as with the speech audiometer or with a good auditory trainer. If not, hearing aid selection is the first goal of the auditory training program.

While specific data must be obtained for each client, it is possible to predict what one will find. If the pupil has normal voice quality one can predict that he will be found to be hard-of-hearing rather than deaf, i.e. his average loss (500 Hz to 2000 Hz inclusive) will fall within the hard-of-hearing range, which is from 30 dB to 85 dB inclusive. His hearing can be expected to respond to amplification. With amplification his aided hearing will be within the normal range, 0 dB to 25 dB inclusive from 125 Hz to 2000 Hz or higher. He will be able to recognize all vowel and diphthong phonemes (male voice) with the possible exception of the high front vowels /i/ and /ei/ and possibly /i/. The second formant frequency for all of these sounds is below 2000 Hz for the average male voice. He should be able to recognize and distinguish among the semivowels /w/, /r/, /l/, and /j/. He should be able to recognize nasal energy although he may not be able to differentiate among the nasal sounds without speechreading, except /m/, with his aided hearing restored to within the normal range, or close to it, up to 3000 Hz. It is assumed that proper medical attention has been secured for all conductive losses that are medically reversible. However, an important reason for hearing testing prior to training is to ensure that there is no conductive component. If one exists it should be reversed before auditory training is initiated.

Professionals have in recent years questioned the wisdom of offering courses in methods of teaching speechreading and auditory training as separate skills inasmuch as vision and audition complement each other and are synchronized in daily living. In fact, it can be argued that they are never (or rarely) taught separately regardless of the intent of the instructor. It is a matter of emphasis. Speechreading instruction (when given with reduced voice) requires attentive listening as well as careful viewing in order to gain the sensory information essential to comprehension. Likewise, in giving auditory training instruction the child or adult is cued both visually and auditorily (look and listen) as to what he is to listen for or listen to before being asked to rely solely on auditory input. In our view, part of any given session should be spent emphasizing vision, part emphasizing hearing, and part combining the two skills for maximum understanding. The emphasis on one mode or another for limited periods of time is to force maximum information. Neither skill should be neglected. Nor should it be assumed that one will learn to speechread naturally or listen attentively unless required to do so. There is ample clinical evidence to the contrary.

This is a practical book. In it we hope to show the reader how to combine speechreading and auditory training in the same teaching session. Our previous book, *Speechreading (Lipreading)**, did not contain "ear-training exercises," nor did it show how many of the materials could be used for both auditory training and speechreading instruction.

An additional purpose of this book is to provide the teacher with an ample supply of materials designed for such instruction. They have been pretested with hard-of-hearing adults and are believed to be both professionally sound and of high interest level. They are to be used with hearing-impaired children and adults who have achieved linguistic competency. The child or adult who has achieved linguistic competency has a basic or inherent knowledge of the grammar of his language. Providing this criterion is met, the degree or extent of the hearing loss will not affect the usefulness of the materials.

What Is Auditory Training?

Auditory training is training designed to improve one's listening habits or skills and, it is hoped, his short term memory as well. For the normally hearing person the goal is improved auditory competency, i.e. gaining and retaining more information through hearing than had heretofore been possible. For the hearing-impaired individual the goal is the achievement of auditory competency.

Auditory competency includes three basic subskills: (1) the ability to recognize significant nonlinguistic auditory events, e.g.

---

*Springfield, Thomas, 1971.

car horn, telephone bell, sound of rain etc., (2) the ability to monitor one's own speech (articulation and voice) so that it does not deviate from normality, and (3) the ability to understand the speech of others. This last and most important skill is called auding.*

Initially, of course, we are dependent on listening. We learn our native language through our ears and are not asked to recognize its printed form until we are about six years old. By the time we have reached the third or fourth grade (eight or nine year olds), if all has gone well, we have mastered reading as a skill. From then on it gradually becomes our chief source of information. Our vocabulary is also extended through reading. We learn to understand the meaning of new words—words that we have never heard anyone say, e.g. picturesque, charisma, etc. As a result we may mispronounce them and say pɪk—ʃɝ—ɛskɪu for pɪk—tʃɝ—ɛsk and tʃɛɚ—ɪzɛm—ʌ for kʌ—rɪz'—mʌ.

Auditory Training for the Normal Hearing

Hearing individuals can profit from auditory training and in some school systems it is a part of the curriculum. Most of us are not very good listeners. We possess only minimal auditory competency. It takes us awhile before we are willing (or able) to give the speaker our full attention. It is probably for this reason that a public speaker starts off with jokes or with material (delighted to be here, etc.) that is not vital to his presentation. Finally when the audience has stopped competing with the speaker and is set to listen he is free to proceed. During the course of his talk he reiterates his major points many times and summarizes them at the end. Auditory memory for most of us is markedly inferior to visual memory.

---

*Auding can be defined as listening to and understanding the speech of others. It is the auditory skill that is comparable to the visual skill of reading — looking at and understanding the printed or written code. If we wish to be more analytic we can define auding as the gross process of listening to, recognizing, and interpreting spoken symbols — speech sounds, words, phrases. Reading can be defined similarly as the gross process of looking at, recognizing, and interpreting written or printed symbols — letters, words, phrases.

Beginning Auditory Training

Beginning auditory training which will lead to auditory competency begins for the normally hearing child in the crib. The infant is, for the most part, self-taught or trained. He gradually learns to associate sound patterns with events (rattle, footsteps, etc. —recognition of significant nonlinguistic events) and then with percepts and concepts (mama, ball, roll the ball, your lunch is ready)—he is learning to aud. The small child gradually masters the grammar of his language and will achieve linguistic competency concurrently with auditory competency. If the child has defective hearing, he will not achieve the necessary goals by himself. There must be intervention. Amplification must be provided. Instruction leading to the achievement of both linguistic competency* and auditory competency must be commenced.

Auditory training for the hearing-impaired begins with hearing testing. Learning occurs during the course of the first pure-tone test. Usually by the end of the first test session the patient will be responding at lower thresholds than initially. He has learned to concentrate and listen for tones which he can barely hear. Provision is made for this phenomena by the routine practice of always rechecking the first thresholds obtained. With very small children auditory training sessions may very well precede an attempt to establish pure-tone thresholds. The child must be taught what to listen for and how he is to respond.

Developmental Stages Leading To Auditory Competency

Following the first auditory test there are four, or at the most five, developmental stages that can be identified in the process of acquiring auditory skills and competency. **Stage** is defined as *(Websters New World Dictionary)* a "period, level, or degree in a process of development, growth, or change."

The stages are: (1) Awareness, (2) Identification—synonyms are recognition and perception, (3) Comprehension, and (4) Retention.

---

*By linguistic competency is meant mastery of the rules of grammar (syntax and morphemes), development of a vocabulary appropriate for the child's age and/or intellectual level, and achievement of the skills (voice and articulation) used in talking.

These constitute the step-by-step goals or products leading to the ultimate goal of auditory competency. Note that discrimination has not been included as one of the stages. It is necessary to distinguish between process and product. A stage is considered to be a product or subgoal. Activities such as *attending, listening, imitating,* and *discriminating* are processes used in the attainment of auditory stages but do not constitute the stages or products. For example, in the process of learning to identify or recognize the given sound pattern for Geneva (one of my names—J.J.), I had to focus my attention, i.e. I had to listen. I had to realize that Geneva was different from other three-syllable words such as elephant—a gross discrimination—and from Genevieve—a finer discrimination. In learning to differentiate Geneva from Genevieve and to recognize Geneva as a distinctive entity or sound pattern, imitation of the respective sound patterns was probably of considerable help.

AWARENESS (of sound). Awareness is the first true stage. "Something is going on" or "I hear it." What we mean by awareness is to know sound exists and probably also its source or from where it is coming. **Awareness** is defined as (Merriam-Webster) "apprehension of an object without active attention to it; conscious of" or (Random House) "having knowledge, conscious, cognizant."

IDENTIFICATION OR RECOGNITION (of sound pattern). These two terms can be used interchangeably if what we have in mind is auditory perception. "I hear it and I know what it is," "That's it" or "It is that." I can let you know I know by repeating it correctly or by pointing to its association—picture or printed symbol. **Recognition** is defined as *(Websters New World Dictionary)* "identification of some person or thing [auditory event] as having been known before or as being of a certain kind," (Random House) "to identify from knowledge of appearance or characteristics" (could be auditory), or *(Roget's Thesaurus)* "identification, cognition, comprehension." **Identification** is defined as *(Websters New World Dictionary)* "an identifying or being identified," *identify* is "to recognize or establish as being a particular person or thing."

COMPREHENSION. The third stage is a sticky word inasmuch as it can also include perception, but it will have to do. In simple terms, it is the "I get it" stage. It has extended meaning for me: affective and cognitive or "catness" as opposed to "cat."

Comprehension is defined as (Random House) "perception or understanding; capacity of the mind to perceive and understand; power to grasp ideas; ability to know" or (Websters New World Dictionary) "the act of grasping with the mind; knowledge that results from this; the capacity for understanding ideas, facts, etc."

RETENTION. The fourth stage is "I understand what you are saying, because I remember what your words mean" and "I remember what a dog sounds like, so I can pretend to bark, etc."

Retention is defined as (Random House) "act or power of remembering things; memory."

Definitions of the processes are as follows:

attention (Merriam-Webster) "listen, take notice, pay attention to, recognize." (Random House) "concentration of the mind on a single object or thought, especially one preferentially selected from a complex with view to limiting or clarifying receptivity by narrowing the range of stimuli." *(Webster's New World Dictionary)* "the act of keeping one's mind closely on something or the ability to do this; mental concentration."

listen *(Webster's New World Dictionary)* "to make a conscious effort to hear; attend closely so as to hear." Random House) "to give attention with the ear; attend closely for the purpose of hearing."

imitation *(Webster's New World Dictionary)* "the act or product of imitating." *imitate,* "to reproduce in form, color, etc., to seek to follow the example of; to act the same; *mimic implies close imitation."*

discrimination (Random House) "to note or observe a difference; the act or instance of discriminating; the resulting state." (Webster's New World Dictionary) "differentiate, distinguish." *Roget's Thesaurus)* "distinction, differentiation, distinguish, separate."

For our purposes *listening and attention are synonymous ac-*

tivities. Note that discrimination is always described as a process; one decides if something is the same or different. If it is different it can be recognized as having an entity of its own.

The stages identified in the development of auditory competency are the auditory rationale for look and listen exercises.

COMBINING AUDITORY TRAINING AND SPEECHREADING INSTRUCTION IN THE SAME SESSION

The answers to "Why do it? Aren't they separate skills?" are largely practical but there are theoretical considerations as well. The child is excused from his classroom for tutoring during certain sections of the day. There is a limit to the amount of time that can be profitably spent in this fashion. Why not include auditory training in the speechreading instruction period in order to ensure that the child becomes an expert listener as well as an excellent viewer. Can he make use of all sensory information available to him? Unless time is set aside specifically for auditory training, it may not occur. The same can be said for adult classes. It may be found to be almost impossible for the busy adult to take both speechreading instruction and auditory training if they do not occur during the same time block.

Another important consideration is that the nature of the instruction makes it possible to use the same or similar materials for speechreading and auditory training. Quick Recognition Exercises and stories, conversation, games, or puzzles are structured and written to promote an increase in conceptual closures.

Auditory competence and speechreading skill are separate skills. The aim of auditory training is improved listening skills so that the hearing-impaired individual gains as much as possible from his damaged hearing. The aim of speechreading is improved viewing habits and skills so that visual information can be integrated with the auditory information and used to complement it. Both skills are aimed at improving perceptual closures. For speechreading, those movements that are highly visible (lip to teeth—f, v; lips puckered—w, hw, r; lips together—p, b, m; tongue between teeth—th) should be recognized instantly. For auditory training those sounds that are heard most easily (vowels, semivowels, and nasals) should be recognized instantly by the majority of the hearing-impaired. The final step, of course, is look and listen—combining vision with audition for maximum information. We believe that the interaction of vision and audition increases effectiveness. The efficiency of each is heightened by the other.

Materials that are useful for speechreading are often also useful for auditory training. Why? Speechreading and auditory training are separate skills which must be taught separately and then combined for maximum understanding. One (speechreading) is concerned with obtaining as much information through the eyes as possible, in order to complement a defective auditory system. The second (auditory training) is concerned with learning to be an expert listener and understanding as much as possible despite a defective auditory system. Both are concerned with reaching perceptual closures (recognition of phonemes and single words). Both are concerned with reaching conceptual closures (understanding the speaker). Quick Recognition Exercises are used for training perceptual closure in both speechread- and auditory training. The difference is in the phonemes selected for recognition and the manner of presentation. There are Quick Recognition Exercises for Speechreading and also Quick Recognition Exercises for Auditory Training.

Auditory Training and Speechreading (Lipreading) Combined As Goals for the Hearing-Impaired

The primary goals of the hearing-impaired person are to understand the speech of others and to be understood by them. The first goal, understanding others, has often been called "auding." It can be defined analytically as the gross process of listening to, perceiving, and interpreting spoken symbols. It is the hearing skill comparable to the visual skill of reading. Hearing loss interferes with auding by reducing the amount of auditory information available to the individual. The greater the sensory deficit, the greater the difficulty the individual will have in understanding both percepts and concepts.

If one is to compensate for a hearing loss he must do so by at least three means: (1) he must supplement his auditory information with visual information; he must learn to recognize visually phonemes which he cannot recognize auditorily; (2) he must sharpen his listening skills and become auditorily more attentive than is "'normal" or usual; (3) he must learn to piece together bits of information and to make "educated guesses" as to what has been said. The hearing-impaired may perceive only parts of the sentence as in telegraphic speech. Telegraphic speech is speech that is incomplete. Small words (is, it, in) and parts of words are often not perceived. Understanding telegraphic speech is comparable to the visual task involved in comprehending cryptic headlines. We know that certain words are missing, words which we subconsciously fill in. For example, "Malpractice Lawyer Fee Curbs Sought" (A group of people is seeking legislation which will curb the size of fees charged by lawyers engaged in medical malpractice suits) or "Workman Band Out to Make a Buck" (The Workman High School Marching Band needs to raise money to finance its activities) or "Many Zonians May Be Seeking U.S. Jobs Soon." (Many United States citizens living in the Panama Canal Zone may be returning to the United States soon to seek jobs.)

In order to anticipate what will be said and to understand when information is missing, one must, of course, be thoroughly grounded in his native language. Fortunately, our language (English) is both patterned and redundant. One can predict the possible words and follow a given phrase or sentence. And fortunately our ideas are also often patterned and redundant. Conversational language is frequently stereotyped—there can be predictors. We talk to each other to convey feelings, to reassure ourselves that we belong, to assure the other person that we like him, to amuse or entertain others, and less frequently, to inform. One can predict the flow of conversation, and fortunately, conversation usually proceeds through association of ideas. One idea leads to another. For example, someone might say, "I had some good halibut for dinner last night." The respondent will not just say "Oh, did you?" and let the topic drop, for this would be rude. There are a limited number of rejoinders—rejoinders which can be anticipated—such as "Oh, did you catch them yourself?" (if talking to a fisherman), "Where did you get it?" (buy it, restaurant), "Nothing better than a good piece of fish," etc. The conversation from then on until the topic is dropped has only a limited number of ways to proceed.

The importance of knowledge of language to comprehension, given limited sensory information, is nowhere more obvious than in contrasting the auding skills of two adults with the same degree and pattern of hearing loss, e.g. 90 dB, one of whom has been deaf since birth and the other whose loss was acquired late in life. The latter will appear to the person used to dealing with congenital losses as having only a mild or moderate hearing loss. His own speech will be normal and he will have little difficulty in understanding others under ideal listening conditions. In contrast, the congenitally deaf individual can be expected to have defective, hard-to-understand speech and considerable difficulty in auding.

ACKNOWLEDGMENTS

It is impossible to thank all who helped me with unfailing encouragement and enthusiasm to complete this book after the demise of Doctor Janet Jeffers. To the many students for whom space does not permit me to list individually and who created materials for this text, please accept my sincere thanks for your contributions.

Much valuable assistance was given by Shirley Oakes, a colleague of ours from California State University at Los Angeles, who edited the important Speech Sound Recognition Test of Doctor Jeffers. This original work would have been lost had it not been published here.

Two who spent hours of their time typing parts of the manuscript must be recognized. My sincere thanks to Evelyn Allan and Lewis Wagman.

I want to add a word of appreciation to Justine Skotnicki who patiently redid the manuscript whenever I changed direction.

It is with utmost gratitude I want to give recognition to Judith Porter, who aided immeasurably in sorting and compiling much of Doctor Jeffers' material. All of Ms. Porter's illustrations are of substantial importance to the text. It was her dedicated collaboration which made possible this final offering.

M.B.

CONTENTS

LOOK, NOW HEAR THIS

Chapter 1

SAMPLE LESSONS

Beginning and Advanced Speechreading and Auditory Training Materials for Children and Adults

1.1. BEGINNING SPEECHREADING AND AUDITORY TRAINING MATERIAL – CHILDREN

1.1.1. Quick Recognition Exercise

Q.R.E. – Visible Initial Consonants

wall	ball	fall
so	though	show

Q.R.E. – Vowel Change

me	my	moo
sew	say	saw

1.1.2. Overlearned Speech – Hide and Seek

Procedure for presentation, see page 69.

AUDITORY TRAINING PROCEDURE: The instructor uses full voice for a second reading. Sentences are chosen at random; the student closes his eyes. He understands by auding and memory. Any sentence not recognized should be repeated with the pupil using both vision and audition.

1. Where are you?
2. Here I come.
3. I see you.
4. Come find me.
5. Can you see me?
6. I'll catch you.
7. Shut your eyes and I will hide.
8. Now I will find you.

9. Are you under the table?
10. I am looking for you.
11. Who is behind the door?
12. Where can you be?
13. Ready or not, here I come.
14. I found you.

1.1.3. Colloquial Sentences with Clue Words

Using three steps for each group of sentences cued by a clue word.

Sentence 1: Look and listen
Sentence 2: Look
Sentence 3: Listen

PROCEDURE. Sentence 1 is given with full voice or slightly reduced voice to assure all understand. Sentence 2 is given with only speechreading. For Sentence 3, students close their eyes, auding only.

Clue Word	*Sentences*
thirsty	1. I'm thirsty. 2. I want a drink of water. 3. I want a glass of milk.
age	1. How old are you? 2. I am five years old. 3. I will be six next month.
name	1. What is your name? 2. My name is John. 3. How do you spell your name?
where to	1. Where are you going? 2. I am going home. 3. I am going home right now.
home	1. We live in a house. 2. It is a big (large) house. 3. It has four bedrooms.
eating	1. Breakfast is ready 2. Would you like orange juice?

3. I would like tomato juice.

fun
1. What shall we do for fun?
2. We could play ball.
3. Let's ride our bicycles.

*1.1.4. Simple Story — A Mouse In My House**

One night I saw a mouse in my house.
I felt sorry for the poor little mouse.
I think it was hungry.
So I left some cheese for the mouse to eat.
The next morning the cheese was gone.
That night I left some cake for the mouse.
The next morning the cake was gone, too.
Every night I fed the mouse.
It was never hungry again.
Then one morning I saw not one mouse, but 2, 3, 4, 5 mice.
Mice were all over my house.
Mice were here.
Mice were there.
Mice were just everywhere!
My mother said I should never, never feed a mouse.
Not in my house!

*1.1.5. A Quiz—What Do You Know About Animals?**

Show the class pictures of the animals named in the quiz. The students should answer each question, giving enough information to indicate they understood all of the description.

1. What animal has big, long ears and can hop, hop, hop very fast? Student–rabbit
2. What animal lives in a tree and says "whoo, whoo, whoo? —owl
3. What animal runs after mice and says, "meow, meow, meow?" —cat
4. What animal chases cats and says. "bow, wow, wow"? —dog

---

*Contributed by Virginia Darrah and adapted.

*Contributed by Maxine Dininny and adapted.

5. What animal gives us milk and says, "moo, moo, moo"? —cow
6. What animal likes cheese and runs away from the cat? —mouse
7. What animal has a bad smell? —skunk
8. What animal runs and plays in the trees and has a big bushy tail? —squirrel
9. What animal is said to be very stubborn? —donkey or mule
10. What animal is fun to ride on? —horse or pony
11. What animal often washes his food before eating it? —raccoon
12. What animal can swing from a tree by its tail? —monkey
13. What large animal likes peanuts and has a big trunk? —elephant
14. What animal carries her baby in her pouch and lives in Australia? —kangaroo
15. What animal has webbed feet and likes to play on the snow and ice? —penguin

1.2. BEGINNING SPEECHREADING – UPPER GRADE LEVEL OR ADULT

1.2.1. Quick Recognition Exercise.

Q.R.E. – Visible Initial Consonants

peak	seek	cheek
thirst	first	worst

Q.R.E. – Visible Final Consonants

waif	wage	ways
moose	booth	boom

*1.2.2. Overlearned Speech – Shopping: Things Said by a Shopper and a Clerk**

1. Let's go shopping.
2. How much is it?
3. What size do you wear?
4. I can't afford it.

*Contributed by Candy Goldworthy.

5. I'll pay cash.
6. Is this cash or charge?
7. May I help you?
8. We're just looking.
9. Where is the fitting room?
10. Buy now—pay later.
11. That store is having a sale.
12. Let's splurge!
13. Would you like it gift-wrapped?
14. It was made for you.
15. Here is my charge plate.
16. I'm broke!
17. We'll hold it for you.
18. Thank you, and come again.

1.2.3. Simple Story — A Fishing Trip

Last week my father, brother, and I went fishing.
We got up very early in the morning.
It was long before sunrise.
We drove about 75 miles to the lake.
We got there just as the sun was coming up.
The weather was beautiful.
We bought some bait and rented a boat.
It was an old rowboat with a motor on the back.
About one-half mile out on the lake the motor stopped.
"There is water in the bottom of the boat," I said.
"It is nothing to worry about," said my father.
"Here is a pail. You bail out a little water and I'll row the boat."
We finally dropped anchor, but I kept on bailing.
"Don't you want to fish?" asked my father.
"No, thanks; I'd rather be sure to stay afloat" was my answer.
My father and brother fished and fished.
I bailed and bailed.
At last they had their limit of fish.
We started for the shore.
"The fishing was great," said the men.
"Let's come again next week."
I'm going to stay home.

1.2.4. Colloquial Sentences with Clue Words

PROCEDURE: Use Look and Listen, Look, and Listen method: See Section 1.1.3.

Clue Word	*Sentences*
vacation	1. We plan to go east next summer. 2. We will see friends in Philadelphia. 3. What is the capital of Pennsylvania?
stories	1. Did you read fairy tales when you were a child? 2. What was your favorite story? 3. Do you remember "Aesop's Fables?"
beverage	1. Will you have cream and sugar in your coffee? 2. Sometimes coffee keeps me awake. 3. So does tea!
home	1. We plan to build a house next year. 2. It will be a ranch-style house. 3. It will be all on one floor.
gem	1. What is your birthstone? 2. The birthstone for April is a diamond. 3. Do you believe diamonds are a girl's best friend?
furniture	1. Her home is filled with beautiful old furniture. 2. Most of it belonged to her family. 3. I like Danish modern style furniture.
camping	1. Our family likes to go camping. 2. Have you ever slept out under the stars? 3. I prefer sleeping in a tent.
exercise	1. Do you exercise every day? 2. I walk 3 miles every day. 3. Sometimes I jog.
telephone	1. Can you hear on the telephone? 2. What is your telephone number? 3. Call me sometime.

1.2.5. *Conversation for Two — Salesman at the Door: A Window-Washing Product**

Salesman:	Hello. Are you the lady of the house?
Housewife:	Yes, I am.
S:	I am selling an amazing new product.
H:	I'm really very busy.
S:	It will just take a minute. It will save you time in the future.
H:	What is it?
S:	It's a spray for washing windows. It will wash a window in two minutes.
H:	How does it work?
S:	(Holding a small spray can) You just spray it on your window. All the dirt comes off and the window dries clean.
H:	I don't believe it!
S:	Let me demonstrate. (Simulates spraying from the can)
H:	This is fabulous. How much is it?
S:	Three dollars a can.
H:	I'll take 3; one for myself, one for my sister, and one for my mother.
S:	Thank you. I know you'll be satisfied. (Salesman leaves)
H:	(shutting the door) I think I was talked into that sale.
S:	(after leaving the house) That one was easy.

1.2.6. *Game — What Helps Us Understand Speech?*

Described are words of four letters. Write each word directly below the one above. Change one letter at a time without rearranging the letter order. When the game is over, a message has evolved. Make sure the first word is understood and written on the board so subsequent words will be correct.

PROCEDURE. A word is described by the instructor. A student

*Contributed by Beverly Ellman and adapted.

volunteers the answer. When all answers have been written on the board the teacher asks, "What helps us understand speech?" If the answer is delayed only the words *read* and *lips* are left on the board. The surprise element adds to the interest of the game. The instructor then chooses a word at random and asks for the description given.

Variation. There can be student response by giving an answer retaining the context but changing the vocabulary used by the teacher.

1. Write a word of four letters meaning what you do to understand a book, magazine, or newspaper.	READ
2. Change one letter in *read* to have a word meaning to be first in a parade.	LEAD
3. Change one letter in *lead* for a word meaning more than one pasture or meadow.	LEAS
4. Change one letter in *leas* for a word which means a smaller amount.	LESS
5. Change a letter in *less* to the name for a girl in Scotland.	LASS
6. Change *lass* by one letter to describe the way a cat drinks water.	LAPS
7. Can you change one letter in *laps* to find the word that completes the message? What helps us to understand speech?	LIPS

A response is required after each word described. This game stimulates an interest in anticipating the possible vocabulary.

1.3. INTERMEDIATE OR ADVANCED SPEECHREADING – CHILDREN

1.3.1. Quick Recognition Exercise

Q.R.E. – consonants in final position

tough	tub	touch
batch	path	pass

1.3.2. Quick Identification Exercise

Q.I.E. – beginning level

moss boss pause (paws)

PROCEDURE: See page 41.

Sentences

1. My father thinks he is the boss at our house.
2. Our dog scratched the door with his sharp paws.
3. Have you ever seen moss growing on a tree?
4. If you pause, it means to wait just a minute.

1.3.3. Story – Smokey The Bear

Introduction (with full voice): This is a true story. It is about a bear that became a legend. He is known all over the United States wherever there are National Forests. Smokey is the best-known animal in our land. He is a symbol for fighting fires.

Clue Words

cub	National Zoo, Washington, D.C.
forester	symbol
clothes	Lincoln National Forest, New Mexico
burned	retired

Exercise Sentences

1. What do we call a bear baby?
2. A forester takes care of our forests.
3. A symbol is something that suggests something else by association. That means Smokey is a symbol for fighting fires.
4. Do you know what it means to retire?

Story Presentation

Smokey the Bear was found as a cub in 1950. He was rescued by a forester after a forest fire. He was found hanging onto a tree in Lincoln National Forest in New Mexico. The poor little bear had been badly burned. The cub was taken to the National Zoo in Washington, D.C. They took care of him until he was well again. He became the nation's symbol against fire carelessness in our national forests. He was called Smokey the Bear. Have you seen a picture of Smokey? He always wears a fire fighter's hat.

He wears blue jeans and carries a shovel. Because of Smokey, people are more careful about fires in our forests. Every year large areas of our forests are destroyed. When Smokey became our fire-fighting symbol, the number of fires dropped. Before Smokey, 31 million acres burned every year. After Smokey, fewer than 3 million acres burned. Smokey was retired. He was sent to the state of New Mexico to enjoy his retirement. He was called a bear senior citizen. He had no children so another cub was chosen to take his place. More than 4 million visitors a year go to see the new Smokey at the National Zoo in Washington, D.C. And the story ends—we hope a Smokey will live happily ever after.

1.3.4. Topic Sentence

SENTENCE. The zebra is an animal belonging to the horse family having brown or black stripes all over a light-colored body.

Variation. Introduce the sentence with a picture in place of a clue word.

Clue Sentences

1. A zebra wears stripes.
2. Some zebras have brown stripes.
3. Others have black stripes.
4. They all have whitish bodies.
5. What does a zebra look like?

1.3.5. A Game — Are You a Good Sport?

PROCEDURE. The teacher uses a term which identifies a sport. The student names the sport.

1. Teacher—What sport would you be playing if the term "touchdown" was used? Student—football.
2. In what sport is the term "home run" used? —baseball
3. What sport would you be watching if you heard "first down?" —football
4. In what game can you earn a "spare?" —bowling

Continue with the same questioning using the following terms:

5. free throw—basketball

6. knockout—boxing
7. slalom or downhill—skiing
8. butterfly—swimming
9. set or love—tennis
10. hammerlock—wrestling
11. jack knife—diving

Let volunteers offer other terms for the class to guess. A variation of this game would be for the teacher to name a sport or game. A student gives a term associated with the sport.

1.4. INTERMEDIATE OR ADVANCED SPEECHREADING – UPPER GRADE LEVEL OR ADULT

1.4.1. Quick Recognition Exercise

Q.R.E. – Obscure Consonant Change

pike	pies	pine
camp	sap	lamp

Q.R.E – Vowel Change Using Front and Mid Vowels Only

jeep	job	germ	jump
lid	led	light	lad

1.4.2. Quick Identification Exercise

win wit rid wind whit

will	rill	writ	wean
weed	read	(reed)	wheat
wheel	real	wait	raid
whale	rate	rail	

1. I hope our team will win the game.
2. He is a funny man. We call him a wit.
3. There is a strong wind blowing from the north.
4. She says she does not care a whit for football.
5. When will I see you again?
6. We must weed the garden today.
7. The wheat should be ripe by August.
8. The boy's bike needs a new wheel.
9. Wait for me.
10. There was a raid on the bank.

11. The gray whale lives in the Pacific Ocean.
12. What is the rate of exchange?
13. We traveled by rail in the good old days.
14. Is that plant (flower) real or artificial?
15. I like to read a good mystery story.

1.4.3. Paragraph for Comprehension — Purring, A Happy Sound

You know you have a happy cat or kitten when you hear it purr. All felines or members of the cat family purr when they are relaxed and peaceful. How does a kitten make that happy sound? It can purr because it has two sets of vocal cords. The true vocal cords a cat uses for growls and communication sounds. When the true cord is relaxed, a second cord flutters with breathing. That makes the purring sound.

Questions

1. Why does a cat purr?
2. What animals purr?
3. Describe the vocal cords of felines.

*1.4.4. Advanced Story — Cactus**

The story of cactus, advanced speechreading, may be given at the intermediate level when introduced with clue words in addition to the drawings. The lesson presented at the advanced level should require only drawings of the cacti for comprehension. Additional visual aids are photographs of these plants found in many *Arizona Highways* magazines.

PROCEDURE: The instructor may reproduce copies of the drawings for each pupil. The orientation is given with full voice. Write the clue words if necessary, go over with full voice then with greatly reduced voice.

Introduction. The word cactus comes from the Greek word "kaktos" (write the word on the board), which means a thorny plant. These spiny plants have lived for millions of years. They are strange plants, and there are many kinds of cacti. In the

*Adapted from *Arizona Highways,* February 1965.

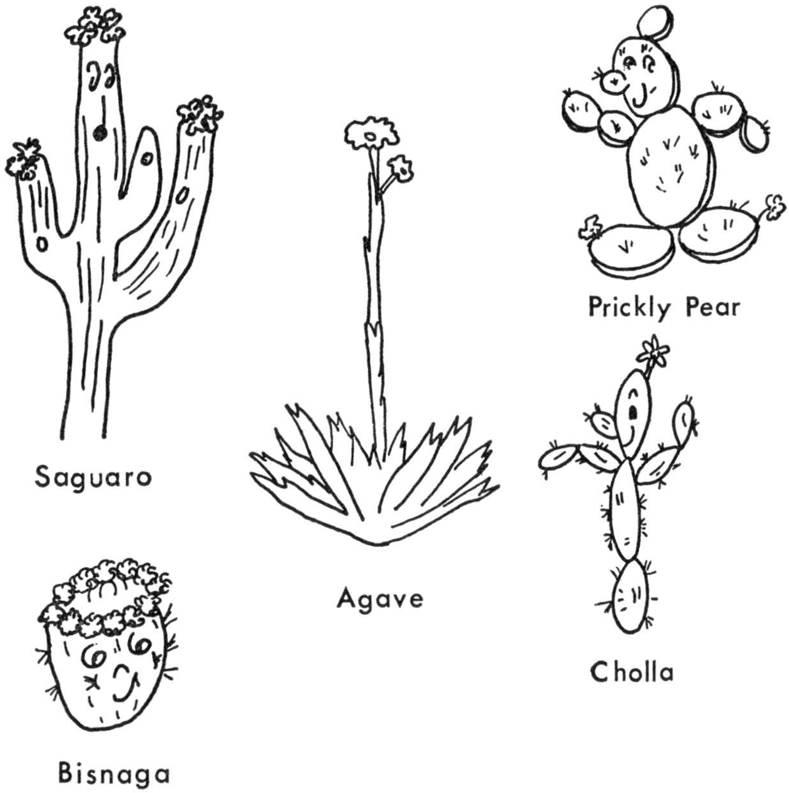

Figures 1, 2, 3, 4, 5.

following story only a few will be described.

Clue Words

survive	root	exotic
adjusted	reservoir	food
conserve	drought	

Cactus plants can live where no others can survive. They have adjusted to their surroundings. They have learned to conserve their moisture. They have developed a huge underground root system. The root system is a reservoir of moisture. The reservoir provides enough moisture for a plant to live through years of severe drought. These unusual plants have beautiful flowers of many bright colors. The blossoms have been described as exotic. Not only are the plants beautiful, they are also valuable. They can provide food for those who live in the desert.

These cacti will be described (write the names and give the pronunciation with full voice):

1. Saguaro (sʌ - ghwa′ - roʊ)
2. Barrel Cactus or Bisnaga (Biz - nɑ′ - gɑ)
3. Century Plant or Agave (ɑ - gɑ′ - veɪ)
4. Two varieties of Opuntia (oʊ - pun′ - tʃjʌ): Prickly Pear and Cholla (tʃɔɪ′ - jʌ)

Saguaro

Clue Words

growth	Indians	caves
sapling	ribs	woodpecker
age	absorbs	elf owl

The saguaro is called king of the desert. This giant plant grows fifty feet high. It grows very slowly and is still a sapling (you might say) at fifty years. It puts out an arm at the age of ninety. It may live two hundred years. The saguaro bears delicious bright-red fruit. The Indians of Arizona are the only people allowed to harvest the fruit. The seeds are ground to make flour. The ribs of the plant are very strong and are used to make shelters. In wet seasons the cactus absorbs much moisture. Then a large saguaro may weigh ten to fifteen tons. There are small caves inside the saguaro. They are caves of small woodpeckers. Every year woodpeckers make new caves. The old ones provide housing for the tiny elf owl. This tiny bird is about the size of a sparrow. The saguaro flower is a creamy white blossom. It is the state flower of Arizona.

Barrel Cactus or Bisnaga

Clue Words

lifesaver	circle	compass
pulp	tilted	candy

Bisnaga is called the lifesaver of the desert. Water may be squeezed from the pulp. This cactus wears a crown of flowers in a circle around its head. It is easy to recognize this cactus because the crown of flowers is tilted, leaning to the south. On many occasions a barrel cactus has served as a compass. It is believed this cactus "enjoys" a long life. Some live well over a hundred years. You can make candy from the bisnaga. It is made much like the candy orange and lemon peel. It is delicious.

Century Plant or Agave

Clue Words

life span	once	ferment
bud	dies	medicine
stalk	tequila (tʌ-ki'-lʌ)	hollow
	pulquey (pul-keɪ)	

How long do you think a century plant lives? It does not live one hundred years. The life span is ten to seventy-five years. The plant sends up a bud twenty feet tall. The cactus looks like a huge stalk of asparagus. It blooms once, then drops over and dies. When the bud is growing it may grow one foot a day. This plant produces tequila. It is made by removing the bud while it is living. The hollow is then pounded with rocks. This makes juices form. When the juice is allowed to ferment it becomes tequila. If the pulpy mess is scraped out of the hollow it becomes medicine. The name of the medicine is pulquey. It is stringy and slimy and does not taste good. But some say it will cure almost anything.

Opuntia: Prickly Pear

Clue Words

grows	eaten	plates
fruit	shortest	

Prickly pear is one type of opuntia. It is known all over the world. It grows in every state except three. These states are Maine, Vermont, and New Hampshire. The fruit of this cactus is very good. It can be eaten several different ways, dried, fresh, or made into a fruit butter. Prickly pear salad is good to eat if you remove the "prickles" first. This cactus has the shortest life span of all cacti. It usually lives not more than twenty years. The blossoms are mostly yellow. Some plants have red and orange blossoms too. The pricky pear looks like plates fastened together.

Opuntia: Cholla

Clue Words

devil	sharp	links
jumping	unpleasant	

The cholla is another opuntia cactus. It has been called unflattering names. Some say it is the devil cactus. Others call it the jumping cactus. It certainly does not jump, but you will! So do not walk too close to the cholla. The sharp thorns will "attach" themselves to you painfully. The fruit is not good to eat. The taste is quite unpleasant. The flowers are beautiful and in almost every color. The cholla looks like links of sausage.

Questions Following the Story (full voice)

1. Which cactus is called the king of the desert?
2. What two animals live in the saguaro cactus?
3. How does the bisnaga act as a compass?
4. How long does a century plant live?
5. What cactus has the shortest life span?
6. Describe what a cholla looks like.

Conclude (with full voice): In the desert wonderland of Arizona, cacti are found in abundance. The riotous beauty of the desert in bloom is an unforgettable experience. The land is protected for future generations to enjoy—don't touch!

1.4.5. A Game of Homophenous Words

A game or quiz to improve visual memory and flexibility.

The teacher defines or describes the first word and gives the letter with which it begins. The letter may be written on the board or given manually if not understood with speechreading. The teacher then gives the category, i.e. bird, insect, or animal, of the second or homophenous word.

Example. Teacher: Write a word of four letters beginning with "L" that describes a feeling of great affection. Beside it write the homophenous word of four letters that is the name of a bird.

(Be sure to allow enough time for the student to write the first word before giving the second description.) The student writes: *love* and *dove*. At the end of the game students may volunteer to write any two of the words on the board giving (with full voice) the gist of the teacher's descriptions.

1. Write a word of four letters beginning with "N" which means close by, not far away. What is a homophenous word that is a wild animal? — *near deer*

2. Write a three-letter word beginning with "A" that is the atmosphere you breathe. What four-letter homophenous word is a small animal with long ears and soft fur? — *air hare*

3. Write a word of four letters that describes what is used to move a rowboat through the water. This word begins with "O." What five-letter word is an animal on whose back you can ride? — *oars horse*

4. Write a word of four letters beginning with "H" that names the part of your arm used when you write. Name a homophenous word of three letters that is an insect. — *hand ant*

5. Write a five-letter word beginning with "V" that describes the speech sounds. What homophenous word of four letters is the name of a bird of any kind? — *vowel fowl*

6. Write a three-letter word that begins with "P." It is a single green vegetable and grows in a pod. What is the homophenous word of three letters that is an insect? — *pea bee*

7. Write a four-letter word beginning with "D" that means the opposite of light. What homophenous word of four letters is the name of a bird? — *dark lark*

8. Write a four-letter word beginning with "R" that is a part of a track a train runs on. What homophenous word of five letters is an animal that lives in the ocean? — *rail whale*

9. Write a seven-letter word beginning with "'M" that is a church in California founded by the Franciscan Fathers. What homophenous word of six letters is the name of a bird sometimes called a dove? — *mission pigeon*

10. Write a five-letter word that describes a very small piece of bread or cake. What homophenous word of four letters is what we call the larva of an insect? —*crumb grub*

11. Write a three-letter word beginning with "W" that means moist or damp, the opposite of dry. What homophenous word of four letters is the name of a small brown bird found all over the United States? — *wet* *wren*

1.4.6. Cross Conversation for Two — Travel

A:
1. Are you planning a trip this year?
2. We planned a long trip last year and had to postpone it.
3. That's what we are expecting to do this summer.
4. We are going by boat so I'll take along some good books.
5. By the way, have you seen the new homes on the west side of town?
6. We may stop at a ranch on our way home.
7. Be sure to take pictures wherever you go.

B:
1. Yes, we are hoping to get away for a couple of months and see the country. What are you going to do?
2. I remember, you were going to Alaska.
3. Will you drive or go by boat?
4. I have just the thing for vacation reading–Sherlock Holmes.
5. The ranch style homes are fine for casual living.
6. There are many good ones all through the west.
7. I will. We bought a new camera just for the trip.

Chapter 2

QUICK RECOGNITION EXERCISES

Exercises for Visual Proficiency

PERCEPTUAL TRAINING THROUGH VISION is accomplished by means of Quick Recognition Exercises. The student is asked to recognize consonant sounds that are highly visible and to gradually increase his closure speed. When he has reached the intermediate/advanced stage he will attempt to recognize the obscure consonant sounds on the basis of vision alone.

Perceptual training through hearing is also accomplished by means of Quick Recognition Exercises for vowels, semivowels (glides), and nasals. The hard-of-hearing person's task is to discriminate among, and to recognize, those sounds on the basis of hearing only.

The introduction of the Quick Recognition Exercises with vowel change are especially designed for the Look-Listen method suggested here.

All exercises are constructed to improve the speechreader's visual and auditory proficiency, flexibility, and skill in arriving at perceptual and conceptual closures. They are classified in this text into five groups: Visible initial consonants for young children, prereaders; Visible initial consonant; Visible final consonant; Obscure consonant; Vowel change.

To explain briefly, the visible consonants for prereaders in Section 2.1 are listed in order of their visibility:

f, v	f, v
w, wh, r	w, hw, r
p, b, m	p, b, m
th	θ, ð
sh, ch, j	ʃ, tʃ, dʒ, ʒ
s, z	s, z

The exercises in Section 2.2, visible consonant in the initial position, consist of two lines of three words. All six visible consonant movements are used in each exercise, one movement per word. The initial consonant movement is varied. The vowel remains constant. The final consonant in each word may be the same or homophenous.* An example of the exercise is:

thank	sank	bank	θæŋk	sæŋk	bæŋk
chin	win	fin	tʃɪn	wɪn	fɪn

The visible final consonant, Section 2.3, has contrastive consonants in that position. The beginning consonants must be from the same group or look alike. The vowel in each word remains constant. Note when the visible consonant is in the final position there are only five used, /f/v/; /p/b/m/; /th/; /ʃ/tʃ/dʒ/ʒ/; and /s/z/. The w hw r become diphthongs in that position. All five movements must occur in each exercise, for example:

gas	calf	cap	gæs	kæf	kæp
reach	reap	wreath	ritʃ	rip	riθ

The obscure consonant movements, Section 2.4, are /t/d/n/l/, /k/g/, and /j/. Note the use of low vowels in these exercises. The mouth is open moderately wide to see tongue movements. Though J is listed as an obscure movement it is not used in these exercises because it is too easily confused with /t/d/n/ and /l/ movements. To complete these exercises /s/z/ are used to give the student practice in distinguishing between these movements where it is possible to do so. An example follows.

*k*ind	*s*ign	*l*ine	kaɪnd	saɪn	laɪn
bal*k*	pau*s*e	bough*t*	bɔk	pɔz	bɔt

This exercise follows a definite pattern. In a two-line exercise of three words the first line contains words beginning with obscure consonants. The vowel remains the same sound,–spelling is out! The final consonant in each word is the same or homophenous.

---

*The word homophene was coined by Alexander Graham Bell to describe words which look alike. The sound pattern in homophenes is different from homophone, or words that sound alike, i.e. homophenes — pay, bay, may; homophones — right, write, rite.

The second line of this exercise uses the obscure consonant in the final position; the pattern is reversed. It can be visualized as:

(1) k. . . ., s. . . ., l. . . .
(2) . . . .k, ...s, ...t(d, /n,/or/l)

The obscure consonant exercise is the most difficult of all Q.R.E.s. The words can be distinguished with accuracy when viewed at close range. An individualized presentation is the most satisfactory. It may be reserved for advanced speechreaders.

For a more detailed description of Quick Recognition Exercises see *Speechreading (Lipreading),* Jeffers and Barley, pages 191-200.

The explanation of the exercises with vowel change has been extended, Section 2.5, for specific auditory training combined with speechreading. They are also devised for rapid recognition but with more effective use of volume, inflection and pitch. The use of low vowels, mid vowels, back vowels, and diphthongs is based on the assumption that amplified hearing is in the normal range from 125 Hz to 200 Hz or higher. High front vowels may not be distinguished in this range and therefore are not included in these vowel exercises.

The vowel exercises are presented with both sight and sound. The first line of an exercise is written on the board. The words are gone over with full voice while the teacher points to each word. Then the instructor repeats the words with no voice or greatly reduced voice. She uses random selection, does not point to the words, and asks the students to respond. Visually the vowel exercises are much more difficult to discriminate. The teacher then asks the students to close their eyes. The words are given with enough voice for correct response. Students with a severe loss may need vision to respond.

The same procedure is used for the second line of the exercise. After both lines have been mastered the pupils work in pairs. Each of the partners takes turns giving the words one line at a time without voice for speechreading. Then each in turn closes his eyes to discriminate by auding. Working in close approximation makes it easier to regulate the amount of voice necessary for every individual. Because of ambient voice noise it is necessary to concentrate more closely on each other.

Again a word of warning. A five-minute practice period is tolerable; longer could be exhausting.

There are four groups using back vowels, mid vowels, back and mid vowels, diphthongs, and back vowels.

The four vowels /u/ʊ/oʊ/ and /ɔ/ are in exercises, in Section 2.5.1, of two lines of three words; for example:

pole	pull	pool	poʊl	pʊl	pul
fawn	phone	food	fɔn	foʊn	fud

The four mid vowels /ɝ/ʌ/a/aʊ/ are in similar two-line exercises in Section 2.5.2, of three words; for example:

curb	cub	cob	kɝb	kʌb	kab
bound	bunt	burned	baʊnd	bʌnt	bɝnd

The back and mid vowels comprise eight phonemes, u/ʊ/oʊ/ɔ/ɝ/ʌ/a/aʊ/. Section 2.5.3 consists of two line exercises of four words each. Two parameters have been added which greatly increase difficulty. The exercises are more complex. There must be discrimination between the greater number of words. Retention is also challenged in the numbers to be received and recalled. A sample exercise follows:

sun	sound	zone	sought	sʌn	saʊnd	zoʊn	sɔt
noose	nurse	nose	gnaws	nus	nɝs	noʊz	nɔz

The four back vowels combined with six diphthongs are u/ʊ/oʊ/ɔ/eɪ/oʊ/aɪ/ɔɪ/aʊ/ɪʊ/. These are also exercises, Section 2.5.4 of two lines with four words to a line; for example:

down	dine	dune	Dane	daʊn	daɪn	dun	deɪn
bowl	bull	pool	boil	boʊl	bʊll	pul	bɔɪl

A group of Quick Recognition Exercises devoted to semivowel (glides) and nasals are included in Section 2.5.5. The semivowels (glides) are /l/r/w/hw/j/. The nasals are /m/n/ŋ/. These exercises are designed for auditory training. They specifically require discrimination among the semivowels and nasals. They are also used for pitch changes. Use three words, each on a different pitch. At times one of the words can be prolonged. As stated before, the hard-of-hearing should be able to recognize these consonant sounds on the basis of hearing only, for example:

might	light	white	maɪt	laɪt	hwaɪt
yea	nay	ray	jeɪ	neɪ	reɪ

2.1. CHILDREN – BEGINNING

These exercises consist of specially constructed words for the young child who cannot read. They should be introduced through the use of pictures, objects, or actions.

PROCEDURE. Start with three pictures, objects, and/or actions (one for each of the first three words in the exercise). As each is shown, the instructor says, "Who can tell me what this is?" After all have responded, continue the presentation in the same manner as a Q.R.E. visible initial consonants, see page 22.

	Exercises			*IPA*		
1.	red	bat	thumb	rɛd	bæt	θʌm
	sock	shoe	foot	sɑk	ʃu	fʊt
2.	boat	run	sit	boʊt	rʌn	sɪt
	this	chalk	fur	θɪs	tʃɑk	fɝ
3.	bird	sack	shirt	bɝd	sæk	ʃɝt
	rain	fat	thread	reɪn	fæt	θrɛd
4.	spoon	fork	mouse	spun	fɔɚk	mɑʊs
	thump	jam	wall	θʌmp	dʒæm	wɔl
5.	sleep	wink	ball	slip	wɪŋk	bɔl
	jump	thing	fun	dʒʌmp	θɪŋ	fʌn
6.	white	sheet	bed	hwaɪt	ʃit	bɛd
	there	sad	face	ðɛɚ	sæd	feɪs
7.	walk	swim	fly	wɔk	swɪm	flaɪ
	milk	that	cheese	mɪlk	ðæt	tʃiz
8.	pail	sand	this	peɪl	sænd	ðɪs
	wash	ship	fist	wɔʃ	ʃɪp	fɪst
9.	boy	thin	soup	bɔɪ	θɪn	sup
	fish	chair	rope	fɪʃ	tʃɛɚ	roʊp
10.	sip	worm	flag	sɪp	wɝm	flæg
	pan	thick	chin	pæn	θɪk	tʃɪn

2.2. VISIBLE CONSONANT MOVEMENTS, INITIAL POSITION–BEGINNING CHILDREN

	Exercises			*IPA*		
1.	pig	wig	jig	pɪg	wɪg	dʒɪg
	that	sat	fat	ðæt	sæt	fæt
2.	those	bows	shows	ðoʊz	boʊz	ʃoʊz
	sail	fail	whale	seɪl	feɪl	hweɪl
3.	thumb	rub	chum	θʌm	rʌb	tʃʌm
	bell	fell	sell	bɛl	fɛl	sɛl
4.	chest	rest	vest	tʃɛst	rɛst	vɛst
	they	say	weigh	ðeɪ	seɪ	weɪ
5.	romp	job	bop	rɑmp	dʒɑb	bɑp
	size	thighs	vice	sɑɪz	θɑɪz	vɑɪs
6.	thaw	saw	paw	θɔ	sɔ	pɔ
	wade	fade	shade	weɪd	feɪd	ʃeɪd
7.	sun	fun	one	sʌn	fʌn	wʌn
	thief	chief	beef	θif	tʃif	bif
8.	wrist	fist	missed	rɪst	fɪst	mɪsd
	those	chose	sews	ðoʊz	tʃoʊz	soʊz
9.	sings	picks	fix	sɪŋz	pɪks	fɪks
	these	cheese	wheeze	ðiz	tʃiz	hwiz
10.	sheet	feet	seed	ʃit	fit	sid
	they	ray	bay	ðeɪ	reɪ	beɪ
11.	shake	fake	rake	ʃeɪk	feɪk	reɪk
	then	pen	send	ðɛn	pɛn	sɛnd
12.	six	figs	jigs	sɪks	fɪgz	dʒɪgz
	third	word	bird	θɝd	wɝd	bɝd
13.	base	race	face	beɪs	reɪs	feɪs
	thump	jump	some	θʌmp	dʒʌmp	sʌm
14.	five	wife	jive	fɑɪv	wɑɪf	dʒɑɪv
	thug	sung	mug	θʌg	sʌŋ	mʌg
15.	their	wear	pair	ðɛɚ	wɛɚ	pɛɚ
	chain	vein	sane	tʃeɪn	veɪn	seɪn
16.	bee	gee	see	bi	dʒi	si
	thin	fin	win	θɪn	fɪn	wɪn
17.	bat	rat	sat	bæt	ræt	sæt
	fair	chair	their	fɛɚ	tʃɛɚ	ðɛɚ
18.	pop	sob	chop	pɑp	sɑb	tʃɑp
	think	wink	fink	θɪŋk	wɪŋk	fɪŋk

19.	four	more	roar	fɔɚ	mɔɚ	rɔɚ
	thick	sick	chick	θɪk	sɪk	tʃɪk
20.	fur	purr	were	fɝ	pɝ	wɝ
	thorn	worn	shorn	θɔɚn	wɔɚn	ʃɔɚn
21.	fox	rocks	jogs	fɑks	rɑks	dʒɑgz
	thank	sank	bank	θæŋk	sæŋk	bæŋk
22.	meat	feet	seat	mit	fit	sit
	though	row	show	ðoʊ	roʊ	ʃoʊ
23.	chew	few	mew	tʃɪʊ	fɪʊ	mɪʊ
	wing	sing	think	wɪŋ	sɪŋ	θɪŋk

BEGINNING ADULTS

		Exercises			*IPA*	
1.	thirst	first	burst	θɝst	fɝst	bɝst
	shine	sign	wine	ʃɑɪn	sɑɪn	wɑɪn
2.	song	wrong	thong	sɔŋ	rɔŋ	θɔŋ
	vain	chain	pane	veɪn	tʃeɪn	peɪn
3.	foal	role	shoal	foʊl	roʊl	ʃoʊl
	ban	than	sand	bæn	ðæn	sænd
4.	thought	sought	fought	θɔt	sɔt	fɔt
	maze	raise	chase	meɪz	reɪz	tʃeɪs
5.	faze	weighs	chaise	feɪz	weɪz	ʃeɪz
	think	sink	pink	θɪŋk	sɪŋk	pɪŋk
6.	thorn	ford	sword	θɔɚn	fɔɚd	sɔɚd
	pack	shack	wrack	pæk	ʃæk	ræk
7.	thus	fuss	muss	ðʌs	fʌs	mʌs
	chide	side	ride	tʃɑɪd	sɑɪd	rɑɪd
8.	wheeze	seize	fees	hwiz	siz	fiz
	thump	pump	jump	θʌmp	pʌmp	dʒʌmp
9.	fall	shawl	wall	fɔl	ʃɔl	wɔl
	theme	beam	seem	θim	bim	sim
10.	things	rings	sings	θɪŋz	rɪŋz	sɪŋz
	sheer	fear	pier	ʃiɝ	fiɝ	piɝ
11.	socks	box	walks	sɑks	bɑks	wɑks
	there	fare	share	ðɛɚ	fɛɚ	ʃɛɚ
12.	jet	wet	vet	dʒɛt	wɛt	vɛt
	thank	sank	bank	θæŋk	sæŋk	bæŋk
13.	chewed	food	boot	tʃud	fud	but
	thing	zing	wing	θɪŋ	zɪŋ	wɪŋ

14.	sank	shank	thank	sæŋk	ʃæŋk	θæŋk
	purse	verse	worse	pɝs	vɝs	wɝs
15.	thinks	jinx	minks	θɪŋks	dʒɪŋks	mɪŋks
	shad	sad	fad	ʃæd	sæd	fæd
16.	firm	germ	burp	fɝm	dʒɝm	bɝp
	then	when	send	ðɛn	hwɛn	sɛnd
17.	thin	sin	win	θɪn	sɪn	wɪn
	Mars	farce	chars	mɑɚz	fɑɚs	tʃɑɚz
18.	theirs	fairs	wares	ðɛɚz	fɛɚz	wɛɚz
	chance	sans	bans	tʃæns	sænz	bænz
19.	sum	mum	thumb	sʌm	mʌm	θʌm
	chase	faze	ways	tʃeɪs	feɪz	weɪz
20.	zest	jest	west	zɛst	dʒɛst	wɛst
	third	fern	burn	θɝd	fɝn	bɝn
21.	thug	rug	puck	θʌg	rʌg	pʌk
	ship	fib	sip	ʃɪp	fɪb	sɪp
22.	chic	meek	reek	tʃik	mik	rik
	thigh	sigh	vie	θɑɪ	sɑɪ	vɑɪ
23.	vein	chain	mane	veɪn	tʃeɪn	meɪn
	thatch	sash	rash	θætʃ	sæʃ	ræʃ
24.	this	fizz	whiz	ðɪs	fɪz	hwɪz
	pierce	cheers	sears	pɪɚs	tʃɪɚz	sɪɚz

2.3. VISIBLE CONSONANT MOVEMENTS, FINAL POSITION CHILDREN AND/OR ADULTS

	Exercises			*IPA*		
1.	catch	gas	cap	kætʃ	gæs	cæp
	worm	worth	worse	wɝm	wɝθ	wɝs
2.	rub	rough	rush	rʌb	rʌf	rʌʃ
	math	mash	mass	mæθ	mæʃ	mæs
3.	love	lump	lunch	lʌv	lʌmp	lʌntʃ
	both	bows	poach	boθ	boz	potʃ
4.	tough	tub	touch	tʌf	tʌb	tʌtʃ
	ham	have	has	hæm	hæv	hæz
5.	dish	dip	live	dɪʃ	dɪp	lɪv
	munch	month	muss	mʌntʃ	mʌnθ	mʌs
6.	cup	cuff	gush	kʌp	kʌf	gʌʃ
	bees	beach	beam	biz	bitʃ	bim

7.	knife	nice	time	nɑɪf	nɑɪs	tɑɪm
	birth	birch	burrs	bɝθ	bɝtʃ	bɝz
8.	reach	reef	weep	ritʃ	rif	wip
	mouth	mouse	pouch	mɑʊθ	mɑʊs	pɑʊtʃ
9.	hump	hush	us	hʌmp	hʌʃ	ʌs
	teeth	leave	deep	tiθ	liv	dip
10.	wipe	wise	wife	wɑɪp	wɑɪz	wɑɪf
	lap	lath	lash	læp	læθ	læʃ
11.	cars	carve	garb	kɑɚz	kɑɚv	gɑɚb
	Dutch	dumb	tough	dʌtʃ	dʌm	tʌf
12.	lap	lath	laugh	læp	læθ	læf
	hitch	his	him	hɪtʃ	hɪz	hɪm
13.	comb	coach	goes	koʊm	koʊtʃ	goʊz
	booth	move	moose	buθ	muv	mus
14.	term	terse	turf	tɝm	tɝs	tɝf
	chef	gem	chess	ʃɛf	dʒɛm	tʃɛs
15.	youth	use	you've	juθ	juz	juv
	mirth	merge	purse	mɝθ	mɝdʒ	pɝs
16.	pulse	pulp	mulch	pʌls	pʌlp	mʌltʃ
	curve	curb	girth	kɝv	kɝb	gɝθ
17.	rope	rose	rove	roʊp	roʊz	roʊv
	each	ease	heath	itʃ	iz	hiθ
18.	as	ash	am	æz	æʃ	æm
	lime	life	lithe	lɑɪm	lɑɪf	lɑɪθ
19.	tease	team	tiz	teach	tim	titʃ
	myth	bib	biff	mɪθ	bɪb	bɪf
20.	tenth	dense	deaf	tɛnθ	dɛns	dɛf
	filch	film	fills	fɪltʃ	fɪlm	fɪlz
21.	gorge	coarse	corm*	gɔɚdʒ	kɔɚs	kɔɚm
	writhe	wipe	rife	rɑɪð	wɑɪp	rɑɪf
22.	lathe	days	dame	leɪð	deɪz	deɪm
	beef	peach	peas	bif	pitʃ	piz
23.	give	kith*	kiss	gɪv	kɪθ	kɪs
	dam	gnash	lass	dæm	næʃ	læs
24.	serve	search	Serb	sɝv	sɝtʃ	sɝb
	soothe	zoom	sues	suð	zum	suz

*corm—a bulb

*kith—friends, neighbors, or acquaintances

25.	edge	hem	ends	ɛdʒ	hɛm	ɛndz
	hutch	hub	of	hʌtʃ	hʌb	ʌv
26.	punch	puff	bump	pʌntʃ	pʌf	bʌmp
	wells	wealth	Welsh	wɛlz	wɛlθ	wɛltʃ
27.	wreath	ream	reach	riθ	rim	ritʃ
	calf	gas	gap	kæf	gæs	gæp

2.4. OBSCURE CONSONANT MOVEMENTS–ADULT AND/OR CHILDREN, ADVANCED

	Exercises			*IPA*		
1.	chat	shag	jazz	tʃæt	ʃæg	dʒæz
	Tom	cob	sob	tɑm	kɑb	sɑb
2.	park	Mars	part	pɑɚk	Mɑɚz	pɑɚt
	cash	sash	dash	kæʃ	sæʃ	dæʃ
3.	bite	bike	buys	bɑɪt	bɑɪk	bɑɪz
	laugh	salve	calf	læf	sæv	kæf
4.	pole	pose	poke	pol	poz	pok
	kite	night	sight	kɑɪt	nɑɪt	sɑɪt
5.	port	pork	boars	pɔɚt	pɔɚk	bɔɚz
	calm	psalm	knob	kɑm	sɑm	nɑb
6.	beg	bell	mess	bɛg	bɛl	mɛs
	sap	gap	tap	sæp	gæp	tæp
7.	rose	rode	rogue	roʊz	roʊd	roʊg
	guess	less	says	gɛs	lɛs	sɛz
8.	guys	nice	size	gɑɪz	nɑɪs	sɑɪz
	razz	rack	ran	ræz	ræk	ræn
9.	bought	balk	pause	bɔt	bɔk	pɔz
	sass	gas	lass	sæs	gæs	læs
10.	chalk	jaws	shawl	tʃɔk	dʒɔz	ʃɔl
	kind	lined	signed	kɑɪnd	lɑɪnd	sɑɪnd
11.	folk	foes	vote	foʊk	foʊz	voʊt
	guest	zest	test	gɛst	zɛst	tɛst
12.	bark	barn	bars	bɑɚk	bɑɚn	bɑɚz
	course	soars	doors	kɔɚs	sɔɚz	dɔɚz
13.	poke	pose	bone	poʊk	poʊz	boʊn
	cab	tam	sap	kæb	tæm	sæp
14.	peg	mess	men	pɛg	mɛs	mɛn
	comb	soap	dope	koʊm	soʊp	doʊp

15.	bag	bass	bat	bæg	bæs	bæt
	goes	sews	knows	goʊz	soʊz	noʊz
16.	gap	Sam	lap	gæp	sæm	læp
	jet	check	chess	dʒɛt	tʃɛk	tʃɛs
17.	shack	shad	jazz	ʃæk	ʃæd	dʒæz
	gourds	towards	swords	gɔɚdz	tɔɚdz	sɔɚdz
18.	fort	fork	force	fɔɚt	fɔɚk	fɔɚs
	cop	lop	sop	kɑp	lɑp	sɑp
19.	shark	chart	jars	ʃɑɚk	tʃɑɚt	dʒɑɚz
	source	Norse	coarse	sɔɚs	Nɔɚs	kɔɚs
20.	mock	mod	moss	mɑk	mɑd	mɑs
	calm	psalm	knob	kɑm	sɑm	nɑb

VOWEL CHART

	Modified for Speechreading and Auditory Training			
	Front Vowels	Mid Vowels	Back Vowels	
	feet i		food u	
High	fit ɪ	fern ɝ	foot ʊ	High
	fate e	ʌ fun	vote oʊ	
	fed ɛ			
Low	fad æ		fought ɔ	Low
		ɑ fond		
		Diphthongs		
	vein eɪ	aɪ file	aʊ fowl, ɔɪ foil, ɪʊ fuel	

Diphthongs have been added to Table II as separate entities. Sounds of diphthongs are more easily recognized as they are visual movement patterns and carry energy power of two vowels.

The diphthong /oʊ/ remains on the chart as a high back vowel because it commonly replaces /o/ in general American speech.

Classification between high and low, front and back, and mid designate the homophenity of the vowels. That is, homophenous high front vowels are /i/ɪ/e/. Homophenous low front vowels are /ɛ/, /æ/. Homophenous high back vowels are /u/, /ʊ/, /oʊ/. Low back vowel /ɔ/ is listed as not homophenous to, nor confused with, the high back vowels or the diphthong /ɔɪ/.

All vowels and diphthongs are grouped and categorized with respect to movement and sound changes.

2.5. VISIBLE VOWEL MOVEMENTS—CHILDREN, BEGINNING

	Exercises			*IPA*		
1.	dog	dig	dike	dɔg	dɪg	dɑɪk
	cat	cut	coat	kæt	kʌt	koʊt
2.	bark	big	book	bɑɚk	bɪg	bʊk
	lick	lack	look	lɪk	læk	lʊk
3.	tip	top	tap	tɪp	tɑp	tæp
	see	say	so	si	seɪ	so
4.	pig	poke	park	pɪg	poʊk	pɑɚk
	tan	turn	tied	tæn	tɚn	tɑɪd
5.	bee	baa	boo	bi	bɑ	bu
	kid	could	can	kɪd	kʊd	kæn
6.	rip	rap	room	rɪp	ræp	rum
	wall	will	wool	wɔl	wɪl	wʊl
7.	big	bag	bog	bɪg	bæg	bɑg
	sun	sand	sound	sʌn	sænd	sɑʊnd
8.	bill	ball	bowl	bɪl	bɔl	boʊl
	key	caw	coo	ki	kɔ	ku
9.	heat	hot	hoot	hit	hɑt	hut
	June	Jane	Jon	dʒun	dʒeɪn	dʒɑn
10.	fine	fan	food	fɑɪn	fæn	fud
	beak	book	bike	bik	bʊk	bɑɪk
11.	seat	sat	suit	sit	sæt	sut
	bing	bang	bong	bɪŋ	bæŋ	bɔŋ
12.	boat	bad	bean	boʊt	bæd	bin
	ten	town	tone	tɛn	tɑʊn	toʊn
13.	knee	now	new	ni	nɑʊ	nɪʊ
	hit	hat	hoot	hɪt	hæt	hut
14.	tick	tack	toe	tɪk	tæk	toʊ
	fee	fie	foe (fum?)	fi	fɑɪ	foʊ(fʌm)
15.	bean	bad	bone	bin	bæd	boʊn
	she	shoe	shy	ʃi	ʃu	ʃɑɪ

16.	pill	pal	pole	pɪl	pæl	poʊl
	boil	pile	putt	bɔɪl	paɪl	pʌt
17.	lamb	limb	loom	læm	lɪm	lum
	team	time	top	tim	taɪm	tɑp
18.	mitt	bat	ball	mɪt	bæt	bɔl
	red	rode	ride	rɛd	roʊd	raɪd
19.	neat	not	note	nit	nɑt	noʊt
	fit	fat	foot	fɪt	fæt	fʊt
20.	pies	pose	paws	paɪz	poʊz	pɔz
	tune	town	tide	tun	taʊn	taɪd
21.	leap	lame	loop	lip	leɪm	lup
	nick	knack	knock	nɪk	næk	nɑk
22.	four	fair	far	foʊɚ	fɛɚ	fɑɚ
	lawn	line	loan	lɔn	laɪn	loʊn
23.	not	nine	note	nɑt	naɪn	noʊt
	loose	lace	less	lus	leɪs	lɛs
24.	teen	turn	town	tin	tɝn	taʊn
	noise	nice	niece	nɔɪz	naɪs	nis
25.	fun	fad	found	fʌn	fæd	faʊnd
	pitch	perch	pooch	pɪtʃ	pɝtʃ	putʃ
26.	zoo	see	saw	zu	si	sɔ
	love	laugh	loaf	lʌv	læf	loʊf
27.	bird	bat	boat	bɝd	bæt	boʊt
	lip	loop	lap	lɪp	lup	læp
28.	barn	burn	born	bɑɚn	bɝn	bɔɚn
	let	lot	loot	lɛt	lɑt	lut
29.	jeep	jam	chirp	dʒip	dʒæm	tʃɝp
	guess	goose	gas	gɛs	gus	gæs
30.	paint	point	punt	peɪnt	pɔɪnt	pʌnt
	girl	goal	gal	gɝl	goʊl	gæl

BEGINNING ADULTS OF UPPER GRADE LEVEL

		Exercises			*IPA*	
1.	lip	lob	lobe	lɪp	lɑb	loʊb
	red	ran	rude	rɛd	ræn	rud
2.	hoof	heave	have	huf	hiv	hæv
	lid	load	loud	lɪd	loʊd	laʊd
3.	sill	soil	soon	sɪl	sɔɪl	sun
	pine	pone	pad	paɪn	poʊn	pæd

4.	tent	tart	toot	tɛnt	tɑɚt	tut
	bought	bat	beat	bɔt	bæt	bit
5.	room	ream	ram	rum	rim	ræm
	sod	soot	seen	sɑd	sʊt	sin
6.	scene	seine	suit	sin	seɪn	sut
	foil	feel	fuel	fɔɪl	fil	fɪul
7.	chore	cheer	char	tʃɑɚ	tʃiɚ	tʃɑɚ
	wind	wand	wound	wɪnd	wɑnd	wund
8.	taught	teen	tat	tɔt	tin	tæt
	hay	how	who	heɪ	hɑʊ	hu
9.	cheese	chose	choice	tʃiz	tʃoʊz	tʃɔɪs
	pour	par	pier	poɚ	pɑɚ	pɪɚ
10.	mode	mad	mid	moʊd	mæd	mɪd
	goat	gait	gone	goʊt	geɪt	gɔn
11.	sick	sack	soak	sɪk	sæk	soʊk
	teal	tall	tool	til	tɔl	tul
12.	burl	bale	pool	bɝl	beɪl	pul
	talk	tick	took	tɔk	tɪk	tʊk
13.	file	foal	fell	fɑɪl	foʊl	fɛl
	meet	mat	moot	mit	mæt	mut
14.	laugh	loaf	leave	læf	loʊf	liv
	vine	van	vote	vɑɪn	væn	voʊt
15.	pass	pause	peace	pæs	pɔz	pis
	knoll	knell	Nile	noʊl	nɛl	nɑɪl
16.	comb	came	calm	koʊm	keɪm	kɑm
	saw	sue	sigh	sɔ	su	sɑɪ
17.	ship	chap	job	ʃɪp	tʃæp	dʒɑb
	bare	bar	boar	bɛɚ	bɑɚ	boʊɚ
18.	ought	eat	out	ɔt	it	ɑʊt
	give	cough	calf	gɪv	kɔf	kæf
19.	zip	sap	soup	zɪp	sæp	sup
	furl	fowl	feel	fɝl	fɑʊl	fil
20.	wax	weeks	works	wæks	wiks	wɝks
	test	toast	taste	tɛst	toʊst	teɪst
21.	firm	fame	fume	fɝm	feɪm	fɪum
	lute	light	laud	lut	lɑɪt	lɔd
22.	geese	goose	gauze	gis	gus	gɔz
	would	wad	wade	wʊd	wɑd	weɪd

23.	hears	horse	house	hɪɚz	hɔɚs	hɑʊs
	beach	batch	botch	bitʃ	bætʃ	bɑtʃ
24.	curve	gaff	cove	kɝv	gæf	koʊv
	dirt	doubt	deed	dɝt	dɑʊt	did

2.5.1. Vowel Movements Using Only Back Vowels—Children and Adults

	Exercises			*IPA*		
1.	pole	pull	pool	poʊl	pʊl	pul
	faun	phone	food	fɔn	foʊn	fud
2.	raw	row	rue	rɔ	roʊ	ru
	goof	cough	cove	guf	kɔf	koʊv
3.	full	foal	fall	fʊl	foʊl	fɔl
	low	law	loo	loʊ	lɔ	lu
4.	pose	puss	paws	poʊz	pʊs	pɔz
	lawn	loon	loan	lɔn	lun	loʊn
5.	tube	dome	daub	tub	doʊm	dɔb
	road	root	rude	roʊd	rʊt	rud
6.	vote	fought	foot	voʊt	fɔt	fʊt
	soon	zone	sought	sun	zoʊn	sɔt
7.	dawn	dune	tone	dɔn	dun	toʊn
	book	balk	poke	bʊk	bɔk	poʊk
8.	tool	toll	tall	tul	toʊl	tɔl
	Shawn	June	Joan	ʃɔn	dʒun	dʒoʊn
9.	root	wrought	wrote	rut	rɔt	roʊt
	mode	mood	Maude	moʊd	mud	mɔd
10.	coat	caught	could	koʊt	kɔt	kʊd
	pawn	boon	bone	pɔn	bun	boʊn
11.	toot	taught	tote	tut	tɔt	toʊt
	goes	goose	gauze	goʊz	gus	gɔz
12.	pooch	push	poach	putʃ	pʊʃ	poʊtʃ
	do	dough	gnaw	du	doʊ	nɔ
13.	shoe	show	jaw	ʃu	ʃoʊ	dʒɔ
	food	foot	fawn	fud	fʊt	fɔn
14.	coo	caw	go	ku	kɔ	goʊ
	dose	dues	daws	doʊs	duz	dɔz
15.	goon	gone	cone	gun	gɔn	koʊn
	bull	bowl	ball	bʊl	boʊl	bɔl

2.5.2. *Vowel Movements Using Only Mid Vowels—Children and Adults*

	Exercises			*IPA*		
1.	curt	cut	cot	kɝt	kʌt	kɑt
	town	turn	ton	taʊn	tɝn	tʌn
2.	wad	word	what	wɑd	wɝd	hwʌt
	bout	but	burn	baʊt	bʌt	bɝn
3.	furs	fuss	vows	fɝz	fʌs	vaʊz
	got	gown	gun	gɑt	gaʊn	gʌn
4.	hurt	hot	hut	hɝt	hɑt	hʌt
	shot	shirt	shout	ʃɑt	ʃɝt	ʃaʊt
5.	mouth	mirth	moth	maʊθ	mɝθ	mɑθ
	was	worse	wows	wʌz	wɝs	waʊz
6.	round	rut	rot	raʊnd	rʌt	rɑt
	howl	hurl	hull	haʊl	hɝl	hʌl
7.	putt	pot	pout	pʌt	pɑt	paʊt
	germ	chum	job	dʒɝm	tʃʌm	dʒɑb
8.	sun	sound	sod	sʌn	saʊnd	sɑd
	found	fund	fern	faʊnd	fʌnd	fɝn
9.	log	luck	lurk	lɑg	lʌk	lɝk
	burrs	bows	bus	bɝz	baʊz	bʌs
10.	one	wan	wound	wʌn	wɑn	waʊnd
	girl	gone	gout	gɝl	gɑn	gaʊt
11.	jot	jut	churn	dʒɑt	dʒʌt	tʃɝn
	loud	learn	lot	laʊd	lɝn	lɑt
12.	lunch	lodge	lurch	lʌntʃ	lɑdʒ	lɝtʃ
	Bert	but	bout	bɝt	bʌt	baʊt
13.	come	cob	curb	kʌm	kɑb	kɝb
	hop	herb	hum	hɑp	(h)ɝb	hʌm
14.	down	done	Don	daʊn	dʌn	dɑn
	birch	pouch	budge	bɝtʃ	paʊtʃ	bʌdʒ
15.	doll	dull	towel	dɑl	dʌl	taʊl
	pert	pond	punt	pɝt	pɑnd	pʌnt

2.5.3. *Vowel Movements Using Back and Mid Vowel Combinations*

	Exercises				*IPA*			
1.	noose	nurse	nose	gnaws	nus	nɝs	noʊz	nɔz
	mirth	mouth	moth	both	mɝθ	maʊθ	mɑθ	boʊθ
2.	doll	dull	dole	duel	dɑl	dʌl	doʊl	dul
	curd	cut	coat	could	kɝd	kʌt	koʊt	kʊd

3.	bunt	burned	bond	bound	bʌnt	bɝnd	bɑnd	bɑʊnd
	yacht	yearn	yawn	you'd	jɑt	jɝn	jɔn	jud
4.	bunk	berg	poke	pock	bʌnk	bɝg	poʊk	pɑk
	round	rode	rude	rut	rɑʊnd	roʊd	rud	rʌt
5.	rock	rogue	rug	wrong	rɑk	roʊg	rʌg	rɔŋ
	firs	foes	vows	fuzz	fɝz	foʊz	vɑʊz	fʌz
6.	down	done	dune	turn	dɑʊn	dʌn	dun	tɝn
	room	roam	rob	rum	rum	roʊm	rɑb	rʌb
7.	sun	sound	zone	sought	sʌn	sɑʊnd	zoʊn	sɔt
	mouse	moose	muss	purse	mɑʊʌs	mus	mʌs	pɝs
8.	shock	joke	jerk	shuck	ʃɑk	dʒoʊk	dʒɝk	ʃʌk
	tune	turn	ton	tone	tun	tɝn	tʌn	toʊn
9.	boom	bomb	bump	burp	bum	bɑm	bʌmp	bɝp
	curl	cowl	cull	coal	kɝl	kɑʊl	kʌl	koʊl
10.	pearl	pall	poll	pull	pɝl	pɔl	poʊl	pʊl
	look	luck	lock	lurk	lʊk	lʌk	lɑk	lɝk
11.	learn	lawn	loan	loon	lɝn	lɔn	loʊn	lun
	come	comb	coop	calm	kʌm	koʊm	kup	kɑm
12.	soup	sup	sop	soap	sup	sʌp	sɑp	soʊp
	gull	girl	goal	cool	gʌl	gɝl	goʊl	kul
13.	purse	paws	bus	bows	pɝs	pɔz	bʌs	boʊz
	fund	fern	fond	phoned	fʌnd	fɝn	fɑnd	fɑʊnd
14.	showed	shot	shout	shirt	ʃoʊd	ʃɑt	ʃɑʊt	ʃɝt
	moose	mouse	moss	muss	mus	mɑʊs	mɑs	mʌs
15.	what	word	wound	wood	hwʌt	wɝd	wund	wʊd
	goose	gauze	goes	curse	gus	gɔz	goʊz	kɝs

2.5.4. Vowel Movements Using Back Vowel and Diphthongs

	Exercises				*IPA*			
1.	whale	wall	while	wool	hweɪl	wɔl	hwɑɪl	wʊl
	boat	put	point	pout	boʊt	pʊt	pɔɪnt	pɑʊt
2.	coot	caught	cute	cowl	kut	kɔt	kɪut	kɑʊl
	full	foal	foul	fail	fʊl	foʊl	fɑʊl	feɪl
3.	pooch	push	poach	pouch	putʃ	pʊʃ	poʊtʃ	pɑʊtʃ
	tire	tear	tour	tore	tɑɪɚ	teɪɚ	tuɚ	toʊɚ
4.	sigh	say	soy	so	sɑɪ	seɪ	sɔɪ	soʊ
	ale	all	owl	oil	eɪl	ɔl	ɑʊl	ɔɪl
5.	dine	down	dune	Dane	dɑɪn	dɑʊn	dun	deɪn
	pool	pull	bowl	boil	pul	pʊl	boʊl	bɔɪl

6.	fume	fame	foam	vibe	fɪʊm	feɪm	foʊm	vɑɪb
	how	high	who	hay	hɑʊ	hɑɪ	hu	heɪ
7.	dial	duel	dole	dale	dɑɪl	dul	doʊl	deɪl
	air	our	ire	oar	eɪɚ	ɑʊɚ	ɑɪɚ	oʊɚ
8.	bake	bike	book	poke	beɪk	bɑɪk	bʊk	poʊk
	soil	sail	soul	Saul	sɔɪl	seɪl	soʊl	sɔl
9.	took	take	tyke	talk	tʊk	teɪk	tɑɪk	tɔk
	goat	guide	good	gate	goʊt	gɑɪd	gʊd	geɪt
10.	mood	mode	might	mate	mud	moʊd	mɑɪt	meɪt
	foot	fought	fond	feud	fʊt	fɔt	fɑnd	fɪʊd
11.	fall	fool	foil	file	fɔl	ful	fɔɪl	fɑɪl
	coos	caws	case	cows	kuz	kuz	keɪs	kɑʊz
12.	should	shoot	shout	shade	ʃʊd	ʃut	ʃɑʊt	ʃeɪd
	raid	round	ride	rude	reɪd	rɑʊnd	rɑɪd	rud
13.	paw	pie	pew	poi	pɔ	pɑɪ	pɪʊ	pɔɪ
	ace	ice	ooze	house	eɪs	ɑɪs	uz	hɑʊs
14.	toy	tie	toe	two	tɔɪ	tɑɪ	toʊ	tu
	gaze	guys	gauze	goes	geɪz	gɑɪz	gɔz	goʊz
15.	lawn	loan	loud	lane	lɔn	loʊn	lɑʊd	leɪn
	butte	bought	bout	boat	bɪʊt	bɔt	bɑʊt	boʊt

2.5.5. Semivowels (Glides), Nasals, and Vowels

		Exercises			*IPA*	
1.	yes	mess	less	jɛs	mɛs	lɛs
	whine	nine	mine	hwɑɪn	nɑɪn	mɑɪn
2.	main	lain	rain	meɪn	leɪn	reɪn
	wheel	yield	kneel	hwil	jild	nil
3.	lamb	ram	yam	læm	ræm	jæm
	rock	mock	lock	rɑk	mɑk	lɑk
4.	you	new	who	jɪʊ	nɪʊ	hu
	mine	wine	line	mɑɪn	wɑɪn	lɑɪn
5.	least	yeast	wheezed	list	jist	hwizd
	rack	lack	nag	ræk	læk	næg
6.	mint	lint	wind	mɪnt	lɪnt	wɪnd
	yak	knack	whack	jæk	næk	hwæk
7.	yacht	lot	rot	jɑt	lɑt	rɑt
	mound	wound	loud	mɑʊnd	wɑʊnd	lɑʊd
8.	lose	use	muse	luz	juz	mɪuz
	rap	yap	nap	ræp	jæp	næp

9.	yell	well	knell	jɛl	wɛl	nɛl
	loan	roan	moan	loʊn	roʊn	moʊn
10.	moon	loon	wound	mun	lun	wund
	rung	young	lung	rʌŋ	jʌŋ	lʌŋ
11.	Yule	mule	rule	jul	mɪul	rul
	law	raw	maw	lɔ	rɔ	mɔ
12.	mean	lean	wean	min	lin	win
	luck	yuk	muck	lʌk	jʌk	mʌk
13.	yore	more	roar	jɔɚ	mɔɚ	rɔɚ
	mend	lend	rend	mɛnd	lɛnd	rɛnd
14.	new	whew	you	nɪʊ	hwɪʊ	jɪʊ
	now	row	mow	nɑʊ	rɑʊ	mɑʊ
15.	yen	meant	lent	jɛn	mɛnt	lɛnt
	mere	rear	near	mɪɚ	rɪɚ	nɪɚ
16.	year	leer	rear	jɪɚ	lɪɚ	rɪɚ
	mile	while	Nile	mɑɪl	hwɑɪl	nɑɪl
17.	Yale	mail	rail	jeɪl	meɪl	reɪl
	wire	lyre	mire	wɑɪɚ	lɑɪɚ	mɑɪɚ
18.	Ute	moot	lute	jut	mut	lut
	rip	lip	nip	rɪp	lɪp	nɪp
19.	yen	when	men	jɛn	hwɛn	mɛn
	walk	lock	rock	wɑk	lɑk	rɑk
20.	wipe	yipe	lime	wɑɪp	jɑɪp	lɑɪm
	lust	must	rust	lʌst	mʌst	rʌst
21.	yard	lard	marred	jɑɚd	lɑɚd	mɑɚd
	meant	rent	lent	mɛnt	rɛnt	lɛnt
22.	whip	yip	lip	hwɪp	jɪp	lɪp
	mole	knoll	roll	moʊl	noʊl	roʊl
23.	lank	yank	rank	læŋk	jæŋk	ræŋk
	nudge	much	rush	nʌdʒ	mʌtʃ	rʌʃ
24.	yawl	wall	maul	jɔl	wɔl	mɔl
	noose	moose	ruse	nus	mus	rus
25.	raw	gnaw	yaw	rɔ	nɔ	jɔ
	week	leak	meek	wik	lik	mik
26.	yearn	learn	word	jɝn	lɝn	wɝd
	gnat	mad	rat	næt	mæd	ræt
27.	new	mew	yew	nɪʊ	mɪʊ	jɪʊ
	worn	morn	lord	wɔɚn	mɔɚn	lɔɚd

28.	yegg (sl)	neck	wreck	jɛg	nɛk	rɛk
	make	lake	wake	meɪk	leɪk	weɪk
29.	nay	yea	may	neɪ	jeɪ	meɪ
	look	nook	rook	lʊk	nʊk	rʊk
30.	you'd	mood	rude	jud	mud	rud
	mare	where	lair	mɛɚ	hwɛɚ	lɛɚ
31.	yawn	lawn	wan	jɔn	lɔn	wɔn
	red	met	let	rɛd	mɛt	lɛt

Chapter 3

QUICK IDENTIFICATION EXERCISES

Materials to Improve Visual Memory and Flexibility

QUICK IDENTIFICATION EXERCISES are designed to improve visual memory and flexibility. It is an important skill. Fifty percent of our language is visually redundant and could be mistaken for something else! The speechreader must retain a visual and audible word, phrase, or sentence long enough to make a rapid shift if his first response is incorrect. To do this he must have an awareness of the homophenity of our words. He must perceive, interpret, and then rapidly arrive at a closure. This is similar to arriving at a correct translation of a foreign language. What was perceived can be reidentified if the speechreader has a good basic knowledge of the appearance of sound movements and patterns.

The exercises have been divided into three levels – Beginning, Intermediate, and Advanced. They are graded with attention to visibility. The Beginning group includes words containing visible consonants in both the initial and final positions. The vowel remains the same in each word. Examples are job, chop, shop, chomp, or beep, peep, beam.

The Intermediate group has words containing both visible and obscure consonants and the same vowel. Examples are pet, met, bet, bed, pent, bent, bend, meant, or feel, veal, feed, feet, field.

The Advanced exercises have visible and obscure consonants and homophenous vowels. Examples are leg, lag, lack, log, long, or jag, Jack, shag, check, jog.

See the Vowel Chart (Table II).

PROCEDURE.

1. The instructor gives any word in the chosen exercise, using very little voice.

2. The pupils are asked to write the word they believe was presented. Do not repeat the word.

3. Each student is asked in turn to give his answer, which is then listed on the board.

4. If all homophenes have not been identified the teacher may say, "Close your eyes; listen carefully. What else could it have been?" The teacher then gives the word using more voice.

5. Any homophenous words still missed are given in sentences by the instructor using a reduced voice.

6. After students respond to the sentences the homophenous words are added to the list on the board.

Variation: Let students choose any one of the listed homophenes and make up sentences.

The total procedure will help the student improve his visual and auditory memory. Gradually he becomes more flexible in responding to the similarity and confusion of homophenous words.

Additional Quick Identification Exercises are listed in *Speechreading (Lipreading)*, Jeffers-Barley, pp.276–278.

3.1. BEGINNING EXERCISES

1. beef peeve
2. bath math path
3. false falls vaults
5. face vase phase (faze)
6. merge purge perch birch
7. sense (cents) says sends sets
8. chip ship chimp gym (Jim)
9. wish which witch rich ridge
10. jam sham jab chap champ
11. whip rip rim rib whim
12. raise (rays) race ways (weighs)
13. bear (bare) mare pear (pair) (pare)
14. march (March) marsh parch barge Marge

15. rinse wince wind winds wits rids
16. match batch patch bash mash badge Madge
17. mum bum bump pump pub pup bub
18. base pace mace bays pays maze (maize)
19. palm balm (bomb) pop pomp bop mop bob (Bob)

***3.1.1.* match patch batch badge Madge mash bash (slang).**

1. There are large patch pockets on my new coat.
2. The policeman wears a badge on his uniform.
3. Will you please mash the potatoes for dinner?
4. I want to find a purse to match my shoes.
5. Let's make a batch of cookies after school.
6. My friend's name is Madge.
7. The party was a bash!

***3.1.2.* palm bob (Bob) mob mop bomb bop pop mom balm**

1. We are going to Palm Springs for a vacation.
2. Did you ever bob for apples on Halloween?
3. I plan to mop the kitchen floor in the morning.
4. The building was destroyed by a fire bomb.
5. He always calls his mother mom.
6. We went to the park for a pop concert.
7. His speech turned the crowd into mob violence.
8. Modern jazz is sometimes called bop music.
9. My grandmother used lemon balm for flavoring in cakes.
10. My brother's name is Bob.

***3.1.3.* wish witch which rich ridge wished**

1. I hope my wish comes true.
2. Alaska is rich in oil.
3. She dressed as a witch for Halloween.
4. Have you ever wished on a falling star?
5. The Blue Ridge Mountains are in Virginia.
6. Which comes first, the chicken or the egg?

***3.1.4.* March (march) parch barge marsh Marge**

1. The month of March has thirty-one days.
2. John Phillip Sousa was called the march king.

3. We went to the marsh to get some cattails.
4. A barge is a flat-bottomed boat.
5. The Indians know how to parch corn.
6. I have a friend named Marge.

3.1.5. mum bum bump pup pump Bub

1. We have had our dog since he was a pup.
2. Be careful – there is a bump in the road.
3. We call my brother Bub.
4. Mum's the word.
5. Can you call a hobo a bum?
6 The boy had to pump up the flat tire on his bicycle.

3.1.6. sense sets sends cents (scents) says sex

1. When I make a mistake I feel like two cents!
2. It says that in the book.
3. He sends her flowers for her birthday.
4. What he says makes good sense.
5. How many sets of tennis shall we play?
6. Can you name perfumes by their scents?
7. What actress is called a sex symbol?

3.1.7. job shop chop chomp (dialect)

1. Do you like to shop for clothes?
2. I like applesauce with a pork chop.
3. My dog likes to chomp on a bone.
4. I am looking for a parttime job.

3.1.8. ship chip chimp gym (Jim)

1. They have built a new gym for our school.
2. His name is James, but we call him Jim.
3. I'm waiting for my ship to come in.
4. We will all chip in for her birthday present.
5. Chimp is a short name for chimpanzee.
6. We bought a used car and it was a gyp.

3.1.9. rip rib rim whim whip

1. There is a rip in his shirt.
2. Will you whip the cream for the pie?
3. The view is spectacular from the rim of the Grand Canyon.
4. I hurt my rib when I fell.
5. She walks in the rain when the whim strikes her.

3.1.10. jam sham jab chap champ jamb

1. My lips chap in cold weather.
2. Be careful or you will jab someone with that sharp stick.
3. The door jam is warped.
4. I like strawberry jam on toast.
5. The boys were having a sham battle at school.
6. Sometimes a horse will champ at the bit in his mouth.

3.2. INTERMEDIATE EXERCISES

1. sad sat sand
2. gash cash (cache) catch
3. latch lash dash gnash
4. bag back pack bang pang
5. sink sing sick zing zinc
6. wheat weed read (reed) wean wheel
7. wit win rid rill will wilt willed
8. fight fine vine vied vile file filed
9. moon mood boot boon pool pooled
10. gap gab gam cap cam cab camp
11. mutt putt bun bud but mud bunt punt
12. pug mug bug puck muck buck bunk punk monk
13. bite might (mite) pine pint pied mine mile pile bile piled mild
14. lap nap nab (slang) lab. lamp lamb tap tam tamp tab dab damp
15. fade fate (fete) vain (vein) (vane) fail failed vale (veil) veiled
16. rain (reign) (rein) wane wade wait weight raid rate wail (wale) whale
17. mitt bit pit pin bin bid mid mint bill mill pill built
18. wide white wine whine rind (Rhine) ride right (write) (rite) while rile riled

3.2.1. gum come cub cup

The initial consonants are homophenous and obscure: /g/k/.
The vowel remains constant: /ʌ/.
The final consonants are homophenous and visible: /p/b/m/.

1. Please come when I call you.
2. I dropped a cup and broke it.
3. Put your gum in the wastebasket!
4. We saw a mother bear and her cub at the zoo.

3.2.2. boot boon mood moon moot pool

The initial consonants are visible and homophenous: /p/b/m/.
The vowel remains constant: /u/.
The final consonants are obscure and homophenous: /t/d/n/l/.

1. My teacher was cross and in a bad mood today.
2. I can't find my other boot.
3. Do you have a swimming pool?
4. Would you like to be an astronaut and fly to the moon?
5. The Boy Scout wore a boondoggle around his neck.

3.2.3. bite bide bind pied pint pine pined might (mite) mind (mined) mine mile pile

The initial consonants in all words are visible: /p/b/m/.
The vowel remains constant: /aɪ) .
The final consonants are homophenous: /t/d/n/l/ and obscure.

1. I am so hungry I could eat a pint of ice cream.
2. Be good and mind your father (and mother).
3. My dog barks a lot but he won't bite you.
4. Do you know the story of the Pied Piper of Hamlin?
5. We have a small pine tree in our yard.
6. If you sprain your ankle bind it up.
7. In what state is gold mined?
8. Our dog pined for us while we were on vacation.
9. Do you walk a mile to school every day?
10. I have a pile of homework to do tonight.
11. We might as well stop this exercise.

3.2.4. lamb lamp dam damp tam dab tab lap nab (slang)

The initial consonants are homophenous and obscure: /t/d/n/l/.
The vowel remains constant: /æ/.
The final consonants are homophenous and visible: /p/b/m/.

1. Mary had a little lamb.
2. The grass was damp with dew this morning.
3. My grandfather is a Scot and wears a tam.
4. I like to watch my cat lap milk.
5. The baby just woke from his nap.
6. We saw the Hoover Dam in Arizona.
7. My sister likes to dab perfume behind her ears.
8. Tap me on the shoulder if I do not hear you.
9. This room should have another lamp for more light.
10. The police will nab the thief.

3.3. ADVANCED EXERCISES (ONLY /ɛ/æ/ɑ/ VOWELS USED)

Exercises 3.3.1. and 3.3.2. are for children, 3.3.3. through 3.3.5. are for adults.

1. test nest lest last lost tossed
2. ledge lash dash gnash lodge dodge
3. web rap (wrap) ram ramp rob romp
4. shed jet shad chat shod shot jot
5. get gat cat cad can cot cod got con
6. fed vet fend fell felt fad fam fat fanned fond
7. gam cam camp cab gab calm cob gob
8. send sent set said sat sad sand sod sot
9. red (read) rend rent wed went when wren ran rant rat rot rod wand want
10. neck deck leg lag lack nag knack tag tack tank dock knock talk
11. led let lend lent den dead debt dent ten tent tend lad tad tat—tan dad gnat lot tot don dot knot (not) nod
12. mend bend bet bed bent pen pet men meant pent bad bat ban pant band pot pond bond pod
13. neb temp deb nab (slang) tab tamp lab. lamb lamp top lob knob

14. dense (dents) tens (tense) tents lens (lends) dens debts nets dance lance lands tans dons tots lots knots (nots) dots nods

3.3.1. rag rack rank rang wreck rock wag whack wok

The initial visible consonants are /r/w/wh/.
The vowels are homophenous, low front /ɛ/æ/ɑ/.
The final consonants are obscure k/g/ŋ/ and homophenous.

1. I think the telephone rang just now.
2. Get a rag and wipe up the milk you spilled.
3. Did you ever have a pet rock?
4. There was a car wreck on the freeway last night.
5. Please put the magazine back on the rack.
6. We gave him seven whacks with a paddle on his birthday.
7. My dog will wag his tail when he is happy.
8. In the army what rank is higher than a major?
9. My mother likes to cook vegetables on a wok.

3.3.2. shag shack shank Jack jag check shock jog

The initial consonants are homophenous and visible: /ʃ/tʃ/dʒ/ʒ/.
The vowels are homophenous /ɛ/æ/ɑ/ low front.
The final consonants are homophenous and obscure: /k/g/.

1. My grandmother sent me a check for my birthday.
2. Sometimes I jog for exercise.
3. The boys built a shack in the back yard.
4. My brother's name is John but we call him Jack.
5. Our dog likes to shag a stick when I throw it.
6. After my father lost fifty pounds he went on an eating jag and gained it all back.
7. Don't touch that wire; you could get a shock.
8. The shank of your leg is between the knee and the ankle.

3.3.3. mood moon boon boot pool put pull bull boat pole mole moan moat bone

Homophenous initial visible consonants /p/b/m/ and homophenous high back vowels /u/ʊ/oʊ/are used.
The final consonants are obscure and homophenous: /t/d/n/l/.

1. Some day I am going to have a sailboat.
2. Did you hear someone moan and cry?
3. I think I will buy some boots and a purse to match.
4. Where did I put my glasses?
5. A mole has been digging up our front lawn.
6. Do you belong to a car pool to save gas?
7. She said she had a bone to pick with me.
8. I'm in the mood for a cup of coffee and a sweet roll.
9. We have a new flag for our flag pole.
10. I hear a siren — pull over to the curb.
11. We went to Mexico to see the bull fights.
12. Have you ever seen a game played in the Rose Bowl?

3.3.4. team deep heap leap tip dip nip dim Tim limb lip tape tame dame name lame

Homophenous initial obscure consonants /t/d/n/l/ and homophenous high front vowels /i/ɪ/eɪ/ are used.

The final consonants are visible and homophenous: /p/b/m/.

1. Whose team won the football game?
2. What is the name of your friend?
3. The water in the pool is eight feet deep.
4. Some do not use much lip movement when they talk.
5. There is a dip in the road ahead.
6. Be sure to look before you leap.
7. He takes a dim view of my opinions on politics.
8. There is a tape measure in my sewing basket.
9. A limb of the tree in our yard broke off in the storm.
10. She is lame and walks with a cane.
11. He offered to give me a tip on the horses.
12. Watch out! That dog will nip at your heels.

3.3.5. let ten net debt lad gnat tan tad tot dot knot lot

Both initial and final consonants are homophenous and obscure: /t/d/n/l/. These are obscure, so this is the most challenging Q.I.E.

The vowels are low front and homophenous: /ɛ/æ/ɑ/.

(Many more words may be added to this exercise within these

limitations, such as lent lend tend dent land dad nod tanned).

1. There are ten women and five men in this class.
2. He is a strong lad for his age.
3. Can you tie a square knot?
4. What is a net ball in tennis?
5. I have a lot to learn about speechreading.
6. Where did you get that beautiful sun tan?
7. Let bygones be bygones.
8. The plane is so high it is only a dot in the sky.
9. What is our national debt?
10. Abraham Lincoln called his son Tad.
11. She is a tiny tot and just learning to walk.
12. Where do all these gnats come from?

Chapter 4

IDIOMS

Idiomatic Expressions to Establish the Semantics of Prevalent Speech

THE RANDOM HOUSE dictionary defines *idiom* as an expression whose meaning is not predictable from the usual meaning of its constituent elements. The use of idiom in the English language is commonly introduced to give color, interest, and often spice (humor) to familiar, colloquial, everyday speech. All languages have their idiom. It is a dialect or style of speaking native to a people. Those from other countries, trained in only formal English, often find the idiomatic structure of our country's language puzzling, just as theirs is to us.

For example: To an Englishman "a ladder in your hose" is "a run in your stocking" to an American. Similarly a Welsh expression "to eat the leek" means "to eat crow" to us. A Spanish idiom is "throw a gray hair to the wind," while we would say "have a ball." A student with a French background in a class of speech-reading was confused when she heard the expression "to come clean" and she exclaimed, "Well, who would come dirty!"

Idiom is a changing language and often reflects the area and times in which it developed. In the eighteenth and nineteenth centuries in America these expressions were considered slang:

a nose to the grindstone
an axe to grind
jump the gun
hang together – credited to Benjamin Franklin

More recently,

behind the eight ball
take a break

Many slang expressions, due to frequent use, become accepted as idiom in general American speech. It is difficult now, however, to think "right on," "out of sight," and "how come" will one day be generally approved as acceptable!

Idiomatic expressions in this text are used similarly to the familiar phrases of Dr. James McDearmon that were introduced in *Speechreading (Lipreading)* by Jeffers-Barley, pp. 211. Because of the obscure meaning of the idiom it is important to give enough information to adequately explain the expression and arrive at a correct closure.

PROCEDURE: The teacher puts an idiom on the board. It is repeated until all respond correctly. A second idiom is added. Both are repeated until mastered. When a third is added, the order of presentation is varied to assure correct response. As many as three or four idioms may be used in one session. The teacher then uses one of the idioms in a sentence.

If the idiom is "up in the clouds" it is insufficient to say, "She has been up in the clouds all day." It must be expanded to give the intended meaning to, "She is so happy daydreaming about her new job she has been up in the clouds all day."

Because of the familiarity of this speech it lends itself to an increased percentage of successful responses. It provides the slow learner and the timid student a chance to feel achievement.

VARIATIONS

1. A volunteer may select an idiom from the board and put it into a sentence for the class to speechread.

2. In a review lesson the instructor asks what is meant by the expressions given in a previous lesson, such as to go halves, up to scratch, sit tight. The review lesson may use optimum auditory input by having the teacher give a review expression with voice while the student listens only. Example: The instructor says, "Do you always go halves and share a candy bar with your friend?" The student responds through auding and memory.

3. Use the literal meaning and ask for the idiom. The teacher asks "What is the expression meaning to be feeling sad and unhappy?" – the answer could be "down in the dumps." "What is meant by 'do not get excited or agitated'?" – the answer might

be "keep cool."

4. A lesson may be introduced with expressions relating to specific categories, such as:

Birds

as happy as a lark
the early bird catches the worm
birds of a feather flock together

Weather

save for a rainy day
be under the weather
take a raincheck

Animals

let the cat out of the bag
to be in the dog house
a snake in the grass

5. Students may bring pictures from magazines illustrative of an idiom. If the picture is not self-explanatory the student may use a sentence to give the meaning.

4.1. IDIOMS

Some familiar idiomatic expressions follow and are used in sentences establishing the gist of the sayings.

A

about face – After they said they would go, they did an about face and refused.

all the same to – If it is all the same to you, I would rather go to the movies next week.

all washed up – When he lost the fight the fans said he was all washed up.

all thumbs – Whenever I try to sew I am all thumbs.

anxious seat, to be on – I've been on the anxious seat all day waiting for him to call.

apple of his eye – Father said his daughter was the apple of his eye.

apple pie order – Her home is always in apple pie order.

axe to grind — If he tries to sell you something be cautious: he may have an axe to grind.

B

backfire — The surprise party backfired when she found out about it.

back talk — All she was getting from her boys was a lot of back talk.

ball, be on the — He is very well informed, always on the ball.

beat around the bush — I want a direct answer; don't beat around the bush.

below par — She is so pale I am sure she feels below par.

be on edge — Fred is so nervous; he always seems to be on edge.

bend over backwards — She always bends over backwards to please her guests.

beyond a shadow of a doubt — The judge said the man was right beyond a shadow of a doubt.

bird, to give one the — He was sent to the principal's office for giving a classmate the bird.

birds of a feather — Those who agree with such silly ideas are birds of a feather.

bite one's head off — I just made a suggestion so don't bite my head off.

blow hot and cold — I can't make up my mind and blow hot and cold about moving to a smaller house.

blow your top — Now don't blow your top until I can explain what happened.

bounce back — After a short rest he was able to bounce back for another game of tennis.

bout with — She is feeling fine after a bout with the flu.

bowled over — When flowers arrived for her birthday she was completely bowled over.

brainstorm — I have a brainstorm; let's stop for something to eat after class.

brass tacks — Let's save time and get right down to brass tacks about the transaction.

break the ice — Fun games are often planned to break the ice at a party.

brush off — She didn't even say good-bye when she gave him the brush off.

by the way — "By the way," she said, "are you coming to my party?"

burn the midnight oil — I have a math exam tomorrow so tonight I'll have to burn the midnight oil.

butter up — Don't try to butter up that teacher; she won't be fooled.

bygones be bygones — Don't fuss about the argument and let bygones be bygones.

C

candle, burn at both ends — He works day and night and is burning the candle at both ends.

ceiling, hit the — Father hit the ceiling when Johnny bent the fender on his new car.

cheek, turn the other — When faced with strong opposition it is hard to turn the other cheek.

chew the fat — They sat up until midnight chewing the fat.

chip on the shoulder — Be careful what you say to him because he always seems to have a chip on his shoulder.

cinch, it's a — I think yard work is hard, but my brother says it's a cinch.

close call — It was a close call but no one was hurt in the accident on the freeway.

close mouthed — He has always been close-mouthed about his affairs.

cloud nine — When the boss raised her salary she was on cloud nine.

cold feet — When Bob got a driver's license he asked me to go for a ride, but I got cold feet and stayed home.

come in handy — A spare house key will often come in handy.

come up with — He always seems to come up with a good idea for making money.

count on — You can always count on him to be on time.
curl your hair — His wild adventures would curl your hair.

D

dash off — I think I will have time to dash off a letter before the postman (mailman) comes.
day, red letter — It was a red letter day for me when I graduated from school.
day, save for rainy — If prices keep going up I'll have a hard time saving for a rainy day.
deadbeat — He never pays his share, the deadbeat!
dog house — He was in the dog house for arriving late for dinner.
dog in the manger — Share; don't be a dog in the manger.
Dutch treat — If we all go to the movies let's make it Dutch treat.

E

eager beaver — He is such an eager beaver he tries to be first in line for football tickets.
earful — If you ask about her grandchild you'll get an earful.
ear, in one and out the other — No matter what I say, it goes in one ear and out the other.
ear to the ground — He always has his ear to the ground for a tip on the stock market.
easy street — He made so much money the family is now on easy street.
eight ball, behind the — She can't seem to hold a job and is always behind the eight ball.
elbows, to rub — She joined a private golf club so she could rub elbows with the wealthy.
ends, at loose — When school is out in June I'll be at loose ends with no homework to do.

F

fast buck — There are some who prefer to make a fast buck rather than an honest one.
fat chance (slang) — You can get me a ticket for the World Series? Fat chance!

fat in the fire — Her angry words added fat to the fire.
feather your nest — She plans to feather her nest with the large bonus she receives every year.
fed up — I am fed up with all those political promises.
feel cheap — He would not give the beggar a penny and afterwards he felt cheap.
feel up to — I don't think I feel up to doing the housework today.
few and far between — I tried to listen but the bits and pieces I heard were few and far between.
fish out of water — I felt like a fish out of water when I wore jeans to the formal party.
fish story — I think he is just telling me a fish story.
flash, in a — Wait a minute; I'll be with you in a flash.
flat-footed — He did not do his homework and was caught flat-footed when the teacher called on him.
fling, have a — He wanted to have one more fling before he joined the army.
fly off the handle — Father flew off the handle when his daughter came home three hours late.
foot the bill — He said, "Let's go to lunch; I'll foot the bill."
foot down — I am going to put my foot down and refuse another piece of pie.
foot, off on wrong — I was trying to make a good impression on my employer but got off on the wrong foot.
fork out — He had to fork out more than fifty dollars to cover the bill.
free as a bird — After her divorce she said she was as free as a bird.
free-for-all —When the baseball player was hit by a pitched ball, it ended up with a free-for-all for both teams.

G

gate crasher — Don't mention the party or there will be sure to be gate crashers.
get away with — That child can get away with anything with his grandmother.
get off one's back — Once and for all get off my back!

give me a hand — Give me a hand with the dishes tonight.
go after — If you want the job, go after it.
goat, to get one's — His remarks are so annoying he gets my goat.
good showing, to make a — The new business seems to be making a good showing.
grain of salt — You have to take everything she says with a grain of salt.
grapes, sour — She said she would not want to go to the party, but we knew it was just sour grapes.
grapevine, heard through — He did not tell us of his promotion; we heard it through the grapevine.
greased lightning — The child won the race going like greased lightning.
green thumb — Anyone who can grow African violets must have a green thumb.
groove, to be in the — That was a great party; everything seemed to be in the groove.
gum up the works — You must follow directions carefully or you will gum up the works.

H

hails from — He said he hails from west of the Mississippi River.
hairs, to split — It is foolish to split hairs arguing the best way to make a strawberry pie.
hale and hearty — Does a big breakfast make you feel hale and hearty?
hand over fist — He made money hand over fist in real estate.
hang up (slang) — She said housework was not one of her hang ups.
hard-boiled — He would give you his last dime but pretends he is hard-boiled.
hard up — They lost a fortune mining gold and now are hard up.
hat, at drop of — Mary will go to a party at the drop of a hat.
hat, keep under — If I whisper something in your ear will you keep it under your hat?
haywire, to go — Everything was running smoothly when suddenly the car went haywire.

head in clouds — When we had our first grandchild our heads were in the clouds.
head over heels — He was trying to keep up with the Joneses and was head over heels in debt.
heads or tails — Her writing is so bad I can't make heads or tails of it.
heels, to cool one's — I had to cool my heels two hours waiting in the dentist's office.
high time — I think it is high time we got together for lunch.
hold out — He said he was going to hold out for a raise or quit the job.
hold water — I am sure his arguments hold water.
hold your horses — Now just hold your horses and speak a little slower!
hook, line, and sinker — He told her a hard luck story and she took it hook, line, and sinker.
hot under the collar — His biased remarks made me hot under the collar.
hot water — The police were looking for him because he was always in hot water.
house, to bring down — Her concert was magnificent; she brought the house down.

I

inch along — There were so many cars going to the parade we could only inch along.
in the pink — She felt in the pink when she heard she had won the prize.
iron out — If we talk it over I am sure we can iron out the problem.
irons in the fire — He works day and night with so many irons in the fire.
itchy feet — Whenever I see a travel folder I get itchy feet.

J

jam, to be in a — She said, "Don't be late for dinner again or you will be in a jam."

jig time – He said he could finish that easy job in jig time.
just so – No matter when you go to her home it is always just so.
just under the wire – We arrived for the opera just under the wire.

K

keep an eye on – I'll keep an eye on your house while you are away.
keep fingers crossed – I think I passed the exam but I'm keeping my fingers crossed.
keep shirt on – Now don't lose your temper; just keep your shirt on.
keep up with – He told his wife that on his salary they could not keep up with the Joneses.
keep your word – You made me a promise, so now keep your word.
kick in – We all had to kick in five dollars for the office party.
kick up one's heels – Let's go out tonight; I feel like kicking up my heels.
knockout – He said, "That new blonde in our class is a knockout."
know the ropes – My job will be easier as soon as I know the ropes.

L

laughing matter – It was no laughing matter when I spilled ice cream on my new suit.
leaf, to turn over a new – I am going to turn over a new leaf this term and get to class on time everyday.
leaps and bounds – When our friends came to help us, the job moved ahead by leaps and bounds.
leave a mark – The basketball coach said, "That superior athlete will leave his mark on the game."
let off steam – It will do wonders for your blood pressure to let off steam.
lick and promise – She said she was in a hurry and gave the housework a lick and a promise.

lie, little white — Have you ever been in a spot where you told a little white lie?

lift, give a — It always gives me a lift to have my hair styled.

limb, out on — I went out on a limb and offered to make all the sandwiches for the party.

line, drop a — Be sure to drop me a line when you are on vacation.

lion's share — She gave the lion's share of her estate to charity.

lip service — Don't give lip service to anything as important as lipreading.

live wire — That child is a live wire and gets into mischief all the time.

long faced — Something is bothering him; he really is long faced.

look high and low — I have looked high and low for my car keys. They are gone!

lookout, on the — She has been on the lookout for a bargain in shoes.

lose your head — In an emergency you don't want to lose your head.

M

make a practice of — He makes it a practice of always being on time for appointments.

makings of — She has the makings of being a good teacher.

man-about-town — He tried to impress us that he was a man-about-town.

man of his word — He is a man of his word; you can depend on him.

mend fences — The politicians come home every year hoping to mend their fences.

mind own business — I was so tired of his advice I told him to mind his own business.

mint of money — Our vacation to Europe last summer cost us a mint of money.

money, to be made of — They must be made of money because everyone in the family has a car.

month of Sundays — Where have you been? I haven't seen you in a month of Sundays.

mouth, down in — He was down in the mouth because he lost the game.

mouthful, said a — She really said a mouthful when she commented on the property tax question.

music, face the — She is over-drawn at the bank and now must face the music.

N

neck, pain in — The waitress said the customer who complained about the food was a pain in the neck.

neck, up to — The boy was up to his neck in homework.

nick of time — She got to school (as the bell rang) just in the nick of time.

nip in bud — Four-year-old Bobby was going to run away but mother nipped it in the bud.

no way (slang) — When he asked for more allowance his father said, "No way."

nose, follow one's — Just follow your nose and you will come to the post office.

nose, lead around by — That woman leads her poor husband around by the nose.

O

odd jobs — He does odd jobs after school to earn extra money.

off-color — He told some stories we felt were off-color.

oil, to pour on troubled water — She is very tactful and is always able to pour oil on troubled waters.

old school — She is of the old school and does not approve of today's mores.

on the fence — I have heard both candidates for the office, but I'm still on the fence.

on the outs — The girl and her boy friend seem to be on the outs after their argument.

on the shelf — If you are a senior citizen don't feel you are on the shelf.

once in a blue moon — I hear from her once in a blue moon.

once-over — That man gives every girl he sees the once-over.

one-horse town – I came from a one-horse town in the middle west.

open and above-board – The executive was open and above-board in his dealing with his staff.

open mind – She is fair and always keeps an open mind on the issues.

out and out – The prisoner told the judge an out and out lie.

out of the woods – She is feeling much better today and is out of the woods.

over one's head – The math problems were over his head.

overplay a hand – He talked so much trying to sell me a car he overplayed his hand.

P

paint the town red – When he celebrated his twenty-first birthday he said he was going to paint the town red.

pass the buck – I asked him for an answer several times and he always passed the buck.

passing the hat – At the finish of the program they planned to gather money by passing the hat.

penny-wise and pound foolish – She saves small change but spends hundreds of dollars on clothes, a penny-wise and pound foolish girl.

pinch, in a – I said I could play bridge in a pinch if they could not find a substitute.

play it safe – On the freeway, play it safe and don't go over the speed limit.

play second fiddle – She left the meeting in a huff when she had to play second fiddle to the chairman.

point blank – He asked her point blank if she would marry him.

pretty penny – My new dress cost me a pretty penny.

pull a fast one – The man on first base pulled a fast one and stole second.

pull rank – The oldest boy likes to pull rank on his young brothers.

pulling a leg – When he said I was beautiful I knew he was pulling my leg.

pumped, being — He asked so many questions I felt I was being pumped.

pushover — The professor is a pushover for pretty girls.

put a stop to — When the teacher walked into the room it put a stop to the shouting.

put on airs — With her newly acquired fortune she tries to put on airs.

Q

question, out of the — When I asked for another week of vacation I was told it was out of the question.

question, to pop the — She said, "I thought he would never pop the question."

quite the thing — At school parties it is quite the thing to wear jeans.

R

racket, to make a — The children made such a racket it made my head ache.

rain cats and dogs — We went for a walk and before we could get home it was raining cats and dogs.

rain check — I can't go shopping with you today but I'll take a rain check.

raise the roof — The boss raised the roof because we took two hours for lunch.

red-handed — After he was told "no more cookies" he was caught red-handed with his hand in the cookie jar.

river, sold down — He was offered a smaller job with the company and felt he had been sold down the river.

round numbers — She always balances her checkbook in round numbers.

run across — I ran across my neighbor in the library yesterday.

runs in the family — They have three gifted children, so brains must run in the family.

S

safe and sound — Our plane flew through a storm but finally landed safe and sound.

salt of the earth – The fine family next door is the salt of the earth.

salt mines – After a long vacation it was back to the salt mines.

scarce, to make self – While they were fighting I made myself scarce and left.

scoop, to – He was a newspaper reporter and always wanted to scoop the news.

scratch, from – She makes all of her cakes from scratch.

see the light – As the parts of the story began to fall in place, she began to see the light.

senses, come to – She came to her senses and decided to save money.

seventh heaven – When he told her they were going to Florida for a vacation she was in seventh heaven.

shape up – The class was told to shape up and quiet down.

shelf, on the – Just because you are a senior citizen it does not mean you are on the shelf.

shipshape – If you leave your apartment shipshape your deposit will be returned when you move.

shoes, heart in – My heart was in my shoes when the car ran out of gas on the freeway.

shoestring, start on a – They have a good business now but they started on a shoestring.

shouting, all over but the – When the score was 35 to 7 we knew the game was all over but the shouting.

shot in the arm – The income tax refund was like a shot in the arm.

shot in the dark – He answered all the questions in the test but some were just a shot in the dark.

sleep like a top – My house-guest said she felt fine and had slept like a top.

slip through fingers – Don't let the chance for advancement slip through your fingers.

small fry – Disneyland is great fun for small fry.

smooth sailing – Now that we have a steady income we should have smooth sailing.

snake in the grass – She had a sweet smile and gracious manner but she was a snake in the grass.

so-so — He said he enjoyed the book, but the movie was just so-so.

soft soap — All those compliments sound like soft soap to me.

sound off — He likes to talk and will sound off on any subject.

spade a spade, to call a — I like to ask her opinion, for you can be sure she will call a spade a spade.

spill the beans — Dont' talk about this or you will spill the beans.

splitting hairs — When she asked about every little detail, the teacher felt she was splitting hairs.

sponge off — He never planned to do anything; he just planned to sponge off the family.

spoon, silver — She has never had to worry about finances because she was born with a silver spoon in her mouth.

square accounts — He breathed a sigh of relief when he could square accounts with his doctor.

stand up and be counted — Don't be afraid to voice your opinion; stand up and be counted.

stitches, to be in — Her funny story had all of us in stitches.

straight from the shoulder — The orthodontist told us straight from the shoulder, "Johnny should have braces."

stretch a point — He would really have to stretch a point to convince anyone that is a new car.

stuffed shirt — He was a bore and a stuffed shirt.

sweet tooth — That pumpkin pie satisfied my sweet tooth.

swing, in full — The party was in full swing by the time we arrived.

T

take a break — Let's take a break and get a cup of coffee.

take bull by the horns — When you have a problem to solve sometimes you have to take the bull by the horns.

talk out of turn — I hope you won't talk out of turn and tell your hostess that mother makes better pie!

talk, small — We were not discussing anything of importance; it was just small talk.

talk, through hat — I don't believe what you say. You are talking through your hat.

teeth, by skin of – We arrived at the airport for our flight by the skin of our teeth.
time, high – It is high time we left or we will miss the bus.
time, kill – Johnny kills time watching television when he should be studying.
thick, laying it on – It is difficult to believe what he says because he always lays it on thick.
throw a fit – A spoiled child will throw a fit to have his own way.
throw in sponge – We've been over this so many times I am ready to throw in the sponge.
thumbs down – The boss turned thumbs down on the employee's suggestion for a raise.
tongue, on tip of – His name is on the tip of my tongue but I can't remember it.
torch, to carry – She broke their engagement but he is still carrying a torch.
track, to get off – When my professor begins to lecture he gets off the track if someone interrupts him.
tracks, wrong side of – Her mother disapproved of her boy friend because she said he came from the wrong side of the tracks.
tree, barking up wrong – I told him we had never met before; he was barking up the wrong tree.
two and two together – Judith put two and two together when she saw her mother hiding a box in the closet and knew it must be a Christmas present.
two bits – Do you remember when a cup of coffee cost two bits?
two cents worth – No one asked me to comment but I had to put in my two cents worth.
two peas in a pod – The twin boys are as alike as two peas in a pod.

U

under the table – He said he had to give something under the table to clinch the sale.
under your nose – Mother said, "Look for it! It's probably right under your nose.
up a tree – If you cannot come for dinner I will be up a tree for a substitute.

upset the applecart — You will upset the applecart if you try to change our vacation plans now.

W

wade through — I have so much homework I'll never be able to wade through it for tomorrow.
walking on air — When I got the good news I was walking on air.
wall, up the — She said the children were so noisy they were driving her up the wall.
wallflower — She refused to go to the dance because she was afraid she would be a wallflower.
wash his hands — The annoyed man announced he would wash his hands of the whole affair.
washout — When he sprained his foot he was a complete washout in the race.
watch her step — The secretary had to watch her step with the new boss.
water, to hold — I am afraid your ideas don't hold water.
water off a duck's back — She never listens to a word of warning. It is just water off a duck's back.
water, under the bridge — Don't fret about yesterday's problems; they are so much water under the bridge.
wet blanket — She would not join any of the games. She is a wet blanket and no fun.
wide berth — When he is feeling cross I give him a wide berth.
windbag — If you keep talking someone is going to call you an old windbag!
winks, forty — You will feel better if you lie down and have forty winks.
wires to pull — He said he would have to pull wires to get that job in Washington.
wool, dyed in the — He is a dyed-in-the-wool politician and will try to convince you to vote for his candidate.
woolgathering — I called your name and when you did not answer I thought you were woolgathering.

Y

yes-man — He is a yes-man and agrees with anything anyone says.

Chapter 5

OVERLEARNED SPEECH

Topic-Centered Everyday Language

Overlearned speech means speech that is heard so frequently that one can anticipate and predict what the speaker will say. These are ordinary and often obvious expressions or statements unrelated in context while maintaining a situational similarity. This is everyday language most people use in "small talk." An example of overlearned speech could be topic oriented as holiday phrases such as:

1. Are you going to a New Year's Eve party?
2. I hope you had a nice birthday.
3. What did Santa Claus bring you?
4. Make a wish before you blow out the candles.
5. We saw fireworks on the Fourth of July.

After the topic is established the listener can expect probable remarks or questions pertinent to the subject.

PROCEDURE: A topic is written on the board. The teacher asks the class to suggest something which might be said about the subject. The instructor then gives the suggested sentences one at a time with pupil response. After all have been given the teacher says, "Now I will give you the sentences while you close your eyes. You have *looked,* now *listen.*" The teacher then chooses sentences at random. Students volunteer to respond.

5.1. BEGINNING SPEECHREADING: CHILDREN

5.1.1. Getting Dressed

1. Let me wash your face.

2. Let me comb your hair.
3. Let me brush your hair.
4. Put on your shirt.
5. Put on your pants.
6. Let mother help you with that.
7. What did you do with your socks? (other sock?)
8. Where did you put your shoes?
9. What dress would you like to wear today?
10. You put your dress on backwards.
11. That's right, pull it down over your ears.
12. Come here, I'll button it for you.
13. Let me tie your shoes.
14. Can you fasten (buckle) your slipper?
15. You must wear a sweater today.

5.1.2. Playing

1. Put your playthings away.
2. Your friend has come to play with you.
3. Let's play hide and seek.
4. Shall we go to the park to play?
5. Would you like to play in the sand?
6. Let's go over to the swings.
7. Pick up your toys.
8. Did you put your tricycle away?
9. You may play after your nap.
10. Is that your toy under the bed?
11. Please come when I call you.
12. Where have you been? I've been calling you.
13. It is time to put your toys away.
14. Oh, you hurt yourself; let mother kiss it and make it well.

5.1.3. Bed Time

1. It's time for your bath.
2. Go jump in the tub.
3. Take a shower and wash your hair.
4. My, you are dirty; let's have a bath.
5. Where did you get such a dirty face?

6. Are you sleepy?
7. Have you said your prayers?
8. I saw you yawn, sleepyhead.
9. Don't you want to go to bed?
10. Are you tired and sleepy?
11. It's time to turn out the light.
12. Good night; I love you.

5.1.4. Eating

1. Wash your hands before you come to the table.
2. Please help mother set the table.
3. You spilled your milk! Don't cry, that's all right.
4. Finish your cereal (breakfast food).
5. Finish your vegetables.
6. Go wash your hands – it's time to eat.
7. Finish your breakfast, then you may play.
8. Would you rather have an apple or a banana?
9. Now you may have some ice cream for dessert.
10. Don't talk with your mouth full.
11. Yes, you may leave the table.
12. Please take your dish to the kitchen.
13. You must not feed the dog at the table.
14. Don't eat so fast.
15. I have a surprise for your dessert – frozen yogurt!

5.1.5. Busy Street

1. Take my hand, we are going to cross the street.
2. This is a busy street, hold my hand.
3. Does the light say go or stop?
4. Don't run across the street.
5. Wait for me. Don't cross the street without me.
6. Come back here. Don't run ahead of me.
7. We must look both ways before we cross a street.
8. Is the light red?
9. Is a car coming?
10. We must walk in the crosswalk.
11. Never cut across in the middle of the street.

12. The light changed to yellow, we must wait.
13. The light is green, now we can go.
14. Wait! That car is coming too fast.

5.1.6. Warning (Parents to Children)

1. Be careful, you'll hurt yourself.
2. Don't touch that knife, you'll cut yourself.
3. Don't go after your ball, you'll get run over.
4. The oven is hot.
5. Don't touch the stove, it will burn your hand.
6. Watch out! Look where you're going.
7. Get off that stool.
8. Don't climb up there, you'll fall.
9. See what happened? I told you not to do that.
10. Put those matches back on the shelf.
11. Don't put that in your mouth, it's dirty.
12. Don't run with that pencil in your mouth.

5.1.7. It's Time to—Things Parents and Teachers Say to Children

1. It's time to get up.
2. Hurry up or you'll be late for school.
3. It's time for breakfast.
4. Breakfast is ready.
5. It's time for you to leave for school.
6. It's time for recess.
7. It's time for lunch.
8. It's time to stop what you are doing.
9. It's time to get ready to go home.
10. It's time for your music lesson.
11. It's time for dinner.
12. Dinner is served.
13. It's time for you to do your homework.
14. It's time for you to go to bed.

5.2. BEGINNING SPEECHREADING FOR ADULTS

*5.2.1. Greetings**

1. Hi!

---

*Contributed by Joal Mayer.

2. How are you?
3. What's new?
4. What's new with you?
5. Where have you been?
6. How's the family?
7. How's the job?
8. You're looking great!
9. You haven't changed a bit.
10. Hello there!
11. Well, fancy meeting you here!
12. What d'you know?
13. I haven't seen you for ages!
14. Welcome.
15. Welcome home, stranger.

5.2.2. Expressions of Approval—Judgmental

1. Bravo
2. Bully for you.
3. Good Boy
4. Good Girl.
5. Atta Boy
6. Atta Girl
7. That's the way to go.
8. That's fine.
9. That's good.
10. That's great.
11. It couldn't be better.
12. That's not bad.
13. Splendid.
14. That's a great idea.
15. That's a brilliant idea.
16. Good work.
17. That's right.
18. That's done very well.
19. Well done!
20. I like what you're doing.
21. That's very good work.

22. That's excellent.
23. Right on.

5.2.3. Telephone

1. The telephone is ringing.
2. Will you please answer the phone.
3. I'll get it.
4. Who is it?
5. I'll call him back.
6. Your line is always busy.
7. I'm expecting a call.
8. You must have the wrong number.
9. Just a minute, I'll call her.
10. Your phone was out of order.
11. I can't hear what you say.
12. I was sorry to miss your call.
13. Call any time.
14. Some people always call at dinnertime.
15. Please call before nine o'clock.
16. Do you have an amplifier on your phone?
17. I always call long distance when the rate is lowest.
18. Cover the mouthpiece of your phone to shut out background noise.

*5.2.4. Days of the Week and Time Expressions**

1. Will you meet me after church on Sunday morning?
2. Will you meet me at six-thirty on Tuesday?
3. I cannot meet you before three on Thursday afternoon.
4. I am so busy I cannot meet you until Friday.
5. I will meet you at four o'clock on Saturday afternoon.
6. I would like to have lunch with you on Friday of next week.
7. I can come for lunch next Monday at one.
8. Will you be home Friday afternoon about three o'clock?
9. Will you be at home on Tuesday morning of next week?
10. May I come to see you on Thursday evening?
11. May I come to see you right after lunch on Friday?

---

*Contributed by Bernice Parker.

12. I am always at home on Wednesday afternoon.
13. I expect to be home every afternoon of next week except Tuesday.
14. I shall be home on Wednesday and Friday afternoons of this week.
15. I will be home every day except Sunday.
16. Monday morning is wash day in our home.

5.2.5. Money, Or the Lack of It

1. Where did you get all that money?
2. How much does it cost?
3. I wish I had a million dollars.
4. I'm not made of money.
5. It's not worth that much money.
6. Where does it all go?
7. That much just for a hamburger?
8. I haven't a dime.
9. You have to pay extra for that.
10. What is it worth?
11. We can't afford that.
12. He makes a good salary.
13. All my change is in my other purse.
14. That costs too much.
15. My taxes have sky-rocketed.
16. The price of meat is out of sight.
17. It's no bargain at that price.
18. I wouldn't pay that much.
19. I should have a raise.
20. Find a penny, pick it up, all that day, you'll have good luck.

*5.2.6. Clerk in Dress Shop**

1. May I show you something?
2. Are you being helped?
3. These dresses are on sale.
4. What size do you wear?
5. This is a size 10, but it runs large.

*Contributed by Ruth Reed and adapted.

6. This is marked down to thirty-five dollars.
7. It is an excellent buy.
8. This came from our better dress section.
9. Do you like this?
10. Why not try it on?
11. The material is wash and wear.
12. I'm sure this will fit you.
13. The color should be good on you.
14. That dress really does something for you.
15. Our alterations are free.
16. Will you take it with you?
17. Is it cash or charge?
18. I think you should try on a smaller size.
19. This is one of the new fabrics and will wash.

5.2.7. Car

1. Do you have a car?
2. What kind of a car do you have?
3. Our car is in the garage for repairs.
4. There is not a scratch on the old car.
5. How many miles do you get on a gallon of gas?
6. We have 75,000 miles on our car.
7. Don't forget to get some gas before you go to work.
8. She never looks at the gas gauge.
9. Oh, dear, my driver's license has expired.
10. Where do you buy gas for your car?
11. My car insurance is due.
12. Do you belong to the Automobile Club?
13. Have you seen any of the new cars for this year?
14. My car wouldn't start this morning.
15. Fasten your seat belt.
16. What kind of a car are you going to buy?
17. Let's go for a ride.
18. Oh, dear, a flat tire!

5.2.8. Traffic

1. The traffic is heavy.
2. Watch out for the traffic.

3. The freeway was jammed.
4. Traffic was slowed down to a crawl.
5. The road was closed to traffic.
6. Heavy traffic makes me nervous.
7. Stay in the slower lane unless you want to pass.
8. Don't be switching lanes.
9. Watch the signal.
10. Traffic was tied up for an hour.
11. There's a detour ahead.
12. Traffic was at a standstill.
13. Have you ever seen such traffic?
14. What do you think is the cause of the tie-up?
15. He should get a ticket for driving so slow.
16. Where do all the cars come from?
17. You need good brakes in any traffic.
18. It took us an hour to get through the traffic at the rush hour.
19. The traffic was slow because of the (fog, rain, snow).
20. I thought we would never get here.

5.2.9. Phrases Used When Back-Seat Driving

1. Watch it!
2. Watch out!
3. Please be careful.
4. Slow down.
5. You're going too fast.
6. I wish you'd keep your eyes on the road while you're driving.
7. You'd better get over on your (right, left).
8. Do you see the car behind us that is trying to pass?
9. The light is green.
10. You just went through a stop light.
11. Can't you drive more carefully?
12. You make me so nervous.
13. You're a mile away from the curb.
14. I'd slow down if I were you.
15. Aren't you driving too slow to be in the fast lane?
16. Do you have to pass every car on the road?
17. I'd rather we took longer getting there and arrived safely.

18. Stay on your own side of the road.
19. Please slow down on the curves.
20. Did you see that stop sign?
21. There's a stop light ahead.
22. You'd better get in the right lane, we're almost there.
23. O.K.! But he's exceeding the speed limit.
24. I think he's signaling for you to move over.
25. Your signal light is still on.
26. Did you signal before you made that turn?
27. What do you mean next time you're going to buy a motorcycle?
28. Don't look now, but there's a cop right behind us.
29. Oh, oh, what did I tell you?

*5.2.10. Getting a Traffic Ticket from a Policeman**

1. May I see your driver's license?
2. Is this your car?
3. Let me see the registration card.
4. Pull over to the side.
5. Do you know what you did back there?
6. I've been following you for three blocks.
7. You went through a red light.
8. You were going ____ miles an hour.
9. Your license has expired.
10. I'm going to write you a citation.
11. Sign here on the line.
12. You should be more careful.
13. This is a one-way street.
14. You were switching lanes.
15. You were driving too slow in the fast lane.
16. Didn't you see the sign saying no left turn?
17. A pedestrian has the right of way in the crosswalk.
18. Sorry! But we can't catch them all!

*5.2.11. Food***

1. I have to shop for some food.

---

*Contributed by Maresa Moliner.

**Contributed by Melody Stouffer and adapted.

2. What do you want for dinner?
3. What would you like to eat?
4. I'm hungry.
5. I'm on a diet.
6. I'm starved for something good to eat.
7. I'll take you out for dinner tonight.
8. We're eating out tonight.
9. An apple a day keeps the doctor away.
10. If there is one thing I love it's good apple pie.
11. I always eat too much when I go out for dinner.
12. They serve too much food at that restaurant.
13. I'm hungry for a steak.
14. Do you ever make clam chowder?
15. She always wants a cheeseburger and a malt.
16. That boy eats too much junk food.

5.2.12. The Airport†

1. What time does this flight leave?
2. I'm so excited about flying.
3. Where is the boarding gate?
4. Have a nice flight.
5. I'm flying first class.
6. Sometimes I get airsick when the weather is rough.
7. I checked my luggage.
8. I've flown many times before.
9. This is my first flight.
10. I like to sit by the window.
11. Your plane is boarding now.
12. Where are you flying?
13. Do you have your ticket?
14. How long does this flight last?
15. Which airline do you prefer?
16. You will have to pay for excess baggage.
17. What time do we arrive in ______?
18. Do you want a window or aisle seat?
19. Which section – smoking or nonsmoking?
20. What movie will they show on this flight?

†Contributed by Nancy Bettenhausen and adapted.

5.2.13. Idiomatic, Hackneyed Expressions of Emotional Stress

1. I nearly died laughing.
2. I almost split laughing.
3. I was bowled over at the suggestion.
4. He had a splitting headache.
5. She was blinded by tears.
6. I was so cold I nearly froze to death.
7. I almost broke my neck to get there on time.
8. The noise nearly drove me crazy.
9. My heart stood still.
10. I fell all over myself.
11. She turned green with envy.
12. He lost his head in the argument.
13. I nearly coughed my head off.
14. The story curdled my blood.
15. I had to bite my tongue to keep still.
16. The child cried her heart out.
17. She broke his heart.
18. She was crushed with the turn of events.
19. I'd give my right arm for a cup of coffee.
20. I had my eye on that chair.
21. Someone is pulling my leg.
22. He must have a hollow leg.
23. We cracked up over the joke.
24. She was so embarrassed she almost sank through the floor.

5.2.14. Forgetful

1. Where in the world did I leave my glasses?
2. Have you seen my car keys?
3. She is always losing her purse.
4. I'll think of it in a minute.
5. My mind is a blank!
6. I can't remember where I put it.
7. Where do you suppose I laid it down?
8. I wish I could remember everything I've ever read.
9. I used to know that, but I've forgotten.
10. Did you remember to turn out the lights before you left?

11. I can't remember his name.
12. I'm sorry — I have forgotten your name.
13. Are you sure you locked the door?
14. I missed my appointment with the dentist.
15. I have a poor memory.

5.2.15. Travel

1. We are going to a ranch this summer.
2. She went to South America last year.
3. Have you been out of town?
4. Where are you going for a vacation?
5. I would like to go through the Panama Canal.
6. They back-packed to the high Sierras.
7. Let's go to the beach over the holiday.
8. They will be gone for about two months.
9. They always go south in the winter.
10. Be sure to take a camera on your trip.
11. We will drive to Alaska in our camper.
12. It would be fun to travel by stern-wheeler on the Mississippi.
13. How far do you plan to drive every day?
14. Next year we are going to New Orleans for the Mardi Gras.
15. If we get a new car we can't afford to go anyplace!

Chapter 6

COLLOQUIAL SENTENCES CUED BY CLUE WORDS

With Expansion of the Look and Listen Technique

THE *Look and Listen* method to introduce colloquial sentences cued by clue words is given in a series of three related sentences cued by one word. The clue word does not necessarily appear in any one of the sentences in that series. The word must be truly a clue to the meaning of the sentences. The three statements or questions related in thought extend information. They provide the speechreader with more knowledge on which to arrive at meaningful closures. The first sentence in the group of three is given with voice. It is labeled *Look and Listen.* The second sentence is introduced with no voice or greatly reduced voice and is called *Look.* The third sentence is given with full voice *while the student closes his eyes* and is designated as *Listen.* The student arrives at a closure through auditory channels and educated guessing.

PROCEDURE:

1. The teacher puts a clue word on the board. Under the clue word she writes *Look and Listen.* Then the instructor says, "I want you to look and listen carefully to what I say. Then someone may tell me what it was."

The first sentence is given with enough voice to assure all have understood.

A student responds repeating the statement.

2. The word *Look* is written under *Look and Listen.* The

teacher says, "Now I will give you a sentence to speechread. Care should be taken to make the sentence as visible as possible.

3. After student response, the instructor writes the word *Listen* under *Look and Listen* and *Look.* She then says, "This time I want you to listen. Close your eyes; let me know if you understand what I say." The third sentence is given with voice. The volume is regulated according to the need of the pupil. When possible, words containing semivowels and nasals should be used in the sentence. If the student has too severe a loss to respond, he should be advised to look and listen for this step. It will relieve him of a sense of inadequacy, frustration, and failure. An aware teacher can tell if he hesitates to respond because of timidity or because of severity of hearing loss.

Many colloquial sentences with clue words in this section have been added without the expansion of the Look and Listen technique. It is suggested the teacher elaborates and develops the sentences to the needs of the pupils. Writing the words Look and Listen, Look, and Listen on the board may be omitted after one or two lessons when the procedure has been established.

VARIATION:

1. A hand signal may be used rather than continually repeating the words "close your eyes." The use of the hand signal helps to maintain the speed and rhythm of sentence presentation.

2. For a second variation no clue word is offered. One or two words in each sentence may be emphasized with *full voice.* The audible stress provides the student with enough information for complete comprehension. For example: "We are planning to *sell* our house;" "When you go on your *vacation* send me a *postcard.*"

Most students require practice to adjust to volume changes during presentation. In a noisy atmosphere a stressed word in a sentence frequently is experienced by the hearing-impaired individual. This kind of exercise (emphasized words) prepares him for these situations.

In the following examples only a few have emphasized words. The teacher will choose those suitable for his students and give one, two, or three stressed words to a sentence.

6.1. CHILDREN

6.1.1. Clue Words: Colloquial Sentences

hungry

look & listen	1. I want something to eat.
look	2. I am very hungry.
listen	3. When will lunch be ready?

raining

look & listen	1. It is raining hard.
look	2. My feet are wet.
listen	3. I wish it would stop.

question

look & listen	1. Where are you going?
look	2. I want to go with you.
listen	3. Let's go to the store.

hurt

look & listen	1. I fell down and skinned my knee.
look	2. It really hurts.
listen	3. Ouch!

crayolas

look & listen	1. I like to color pictures.
look	2. I will make a picture for you.
listen	3. Where are my crayons?

more

look & listen	1. May I have another cookie?
look	2. I want a glass of milk too.
listen	3. The milk is all gone.

hurry

look & listen	1. Hurry or you will be late for school.
look	2. Where are your shoes?
listen	3. Here is your sweater.

6.1.2. Clue Words: Colloquial Sentences

red

look & listen	1. The apple is red.
look	2. I like apples.
listen	3. I want a red apple now.

yellow

look & listen	1. A banana is yellow.
look	2. A sunflower is yellow.
listen	3. A ripe lemon is yellow.

orange

look & listen	1. A pumpkin is orange.
look	2. A persimmon is orange.
listen	3. An orange is orange, too.

white

look & listen	1. The cloud in the sky is white.
look	2. Snow is white.
listen	3. I have a white kitten.

blue

look & listen	1. Point to the blue sky.
look	2. My eyes are blue.
listen	3. I like to eat blueberries.

green

look & listen	1. The grass is green.
look	2. I like green grapes.
listen	3. Do you like a green salad?

brown

look & listen	1. My new shoes are brown.
look	2. I have a brown sweater too.
listen	3. Chocolate candy is brown.

purple

look & listen	1. I had purple grapes for lunch.
look	2. Purple grape juice is good.
listen	3. We have purple pansies in our yard.

6.1.3. Clue Word: Colloquial Sentences

doll

look & listen	1. I have a new doll.
look	2. I like to comb her hair.
listen	3. My doll says "ma-ma."

wagon

look & listen	1. I have a red wagon.

look	2. Give me a ride in my wagon.
listen	3. Then I'll give you a ride.
tricycle	
look & listen	1. My sister has a tricycle.
look	2. She got it for her birthday.
listen	3. She wants to ride it all the time.
ball	
look & listen	1. Let's play baseball.
look	2. We can play after school.
listen	3. Do you have a baseball mitt?
football	
look & listen	1. Have you seen my football?
look	2. My brother gave it to me.
listen	3. Maybe I left it at your house.
kite	
look & listen	1. I fly my kite when the wind blows.
look	2. The wind is blowing today.
listen	3. Let's go to the park to fly our kites.
roller skate	
look & listen	1. Do you have roller skates?
look	2. When my skates go fast I fall down.
listen	3. Sometimes that hurts.
bean bag	
look & listen	1. We play with bean bags at school.
look	2. Throw the bean bag to me.
listen	3. Not so fast!

6.1.4. Clue Words: Colloquial Sentences

animal	1. My friend has a hamster for a pet.
	2. Do you have a pet?
	3. I would like a white rat for a pet.
weather	1. Did you hear it rain last night?
	2. It poured.
	3. The lightning and thunder woke me.
vacation	1. He is going to a camp in the mountains this summer.
	2. It is a Boy Scout camp.

	3. I would like to go too.
movie	1. I wish I could go to a show tonight.
	2. I like movies about animals.
	3. My mother says no movies on school nights.
lesson	1. I have to practice my music lesson.
	2. Can you play the piano?
	3. I would like to play drums.
picnic	1. We had all the hot dogs we could eat.
	2. I ate seven hot dogs.
	3. Then I had a stomach ache.
time	1. We can go home in fifteen minutes.
	2. That clock must be slow.
	3. No more school until Monday.
company	1. We had company and I had to sleep on the floor.
	2. It was fun.
	3. My dog slept with me.

6.1.5. Clue Words: Colloquial Sentences

buying	1. I like to go shopping with my mother.
movie	2. Have you seen a movie about Lassie?
old	3. My shoes are worn out.
growing	4. My feet are too big for my shoes.
helpful	5. I like my new hearing aid.
play	6. I like to play in the snow.
snow	7. We made a snowman.
angel	8. Do you know how to make an angel in the snow?
hunter	9. Our cat caught a mouse.
dress	10. Can you tie your shoes?
sweater	11. Where is my warm sweater?
full	12. I ate too much lunch.

6.1.6. Clue Words: Colloquial Sentences

walk	1. I had to walk to school this morning.
late	2. I missed the bus.
age	3. My birthday is next month.

dessert	4. We had pumpkin pie for dinner.
draw	5. I like to draw pictures.
hurt	6. How did you get that bruise on your arm?
zoo	7. We are going to see some animals tomorrow.
spelling	8. How many words did you miss?
homework	9. I have to do my homework before I can play.
dress	10. I like your new dress.

6.1.7. Clue Words: Colloquial Sentences:

animals	1. Have you ever gone to a zoo?
envy	2. I wish I could whistle like you do.
accident	3. He fell down and got a bump on his head.
reward	4. The man gave me a dollar when I found his wallet.
music	5. My father plays a guitar.
holiday	6. There will be no school next Monday.
exercise	7. Let's roller skate after school.
funnies	8. I like to read the comics.
noon	9. It's time for lunch.
barefoot	10. I like to take my shoes and socks off and walk in the mud.

6.1.8. Clue Words: Colloquial Sentences

game	1. I like to play baseball.
lost	2. My dog ran away.
clock	3. It is time to go to school.
eat	4. I wish I could have a hamburger.
visit	5. We are going to see my grandmother.
run	6. Hurry or you'll be late.
car	7. My father bought a Ford.
age	8. How old are you?
raining	9. Don't forget your raincoat.
smile	10. Do you like to have your picture taken?

6.1.9. Clue Words: Colloquial Sentences

pet	1. I have a dog and his name is Bowser.
rain	2. I like to hear the rain on the roof.

present	3. I brought an apple for the teacher.
story	4. Do you like fairy tales?
favorite	5. I like chocolate ice cream the best of all.
tardy	6. She was late for school this morning.
country	7. Would you like to live on a farm?
happy	8. Our baby laughed when I made a face.
bike	9. He has a new ten-speed bicycle.
playground	10. We have swings and slides to play on at school.

6.1.10.

Clue Words:	*Colloquial Sentences*
parade	1. We watched the Rose Parade on TV.
pool	2. We are taking swimming lessons.
scowling	3. Are you mad at me?
sport	4. I am going to the football game Saturday with my father.
smile	5. Let's see a happy face.
holiday	6. Oh boy—no school next week.
afraid?	7. I saw a mouse in the garage yesterday.
TV	8. Do you like to watch the cartoons?
game	9. What is your favorite sport?
food	10. Do you ever eat pizza?
movie	11. We saw a movie at school today.
broke	12. I spent all my allowance for this week.

6.1.11.

Clue Words:	*Colloquial Sentences*
wet	1. Let's get in out of the rain.
trip	2. We are going camping this weekend.
nervous	3. What makes you so jumpy?
eat	4. What are you going to have for dinner tonight?
sad	5. Don't cry!
happy	6. I'm sure glad she's smiling today.
present	7. She got a watch for her birthday.
weary	8. Are you tired?
siren	9. Where's the fire?
exercise	10. My father jogs three miles a day.

picnic	11. We took our lunch and went to the park.
reward	12. My brother was made an Eagle Scout.

6.1.12. Clue Words: Colloquial Sentences

time	1. How long does it take you to get to school?
movie	2. Would you like to go to a show tonight?
whiskers	3. Many of our presidents have worn beards.
hurry	4. We had to run for the bus this morning.
sick	5. She has been out of school with a cold.
moving	6. We are going to move to a new home.
misplaced	7. Where did I put my homework?
game	8. Baseball is the number one sport in Japan and the United States.
talking	9. Were you speaking to me?
more	10. Would you like another piece of pie?
gloves	11. Mittens keep my hands warm when it is cold.
hot	12. It is too warm to wear a sweater today.

6.1.13. Clue Words: Colloquial Sentences

fat	1. My father says he is going on a diet.
cold	2. It is cold outside.
weiners	3. I had two hot dogs in my lunch.
memory	4. Do you remember your first day of school?
safe	5. We have seat belts in our car.
naughty	6. My baby brother won't eat vegetables.
pills	7. We take vitamins every morning.
too bad!	8. The rain spoiled the ball game.
job	9. My father is a fireman.
swim	10. My dog likes to paddle in the water.
practices	11. My sister plays the piano every day.
dog laws	12. If you walk the dog be sure he is on a leash.
boo!	13. He dressed like a ghost to scare us on Halloween.

6.1.14. Clue Words: Colloquial Sentences

paper	1. As soon as the (name of paper) comes I look at the comics.

soup	2.	My mother makes good clam chowder.
make a wish	3.	Did you ever wish on a falling star?
party	4.	We are going to have a surprise birthday party for my sister.
music	5.	I want to play the guitar when I grow up.
same	6.	John and James are identical twins.
rain	7.	Look! It is pouring and I don't have a coat.
gift	8.	I bought my father a fishing rod for Christmas.
burn	9.	I stayed in the sun too long and got a sunburn.
distance	10.	How far can you throw a ball?

6.1.15. Clue Words: Colloquial Sentences

time	1.	My watch is five minutes fast.
magazine	2.	I like the pictures in the *National Geographic.*
funny	3.	We laughed at the clowns in the circus.
baseball	4.	Have you ever seen a World Series game?
dessert	5.	We had strawberry shortcake for dessert.
sleepy	6.	Are you tired? I just saw you yawn.
food	7.	We had hamburgers, potato chips, and ice cream at the picnic.
math	8.	I had a mistake on my arithmetic paper.
hungry	9.	That boy is always asking for something to eat.
pilot	10.	I would like to fly an airplane when I grow up.
ouch!	11.	I hit my thumb with a hammer.

6.1.16. Clue Words: Colloquial Sentences

vacation	1.	We go to my grandfather's farm every summer.
storm	2.	She is afraid of thunder and lightning.
away	3.	Where were you yesterday?
dentist	4.	I have never had a tooth filled.
alike	5.	You look just like your big brother.

question	6. What shall we do?
library	7. We have to be very quiet in the library.
danger	8. Do not play in the street.
call me	9. What is your telephone number?
fun	10. Let's ride our bicycles.

6.1.17. Clue Words: Colloquial Sentences

starved	1. I am so hungry.
remember	2. Don't forget your homework.
bus	3. Some of my friends ride to school every day.
Cub Scouts	4. My troop is going camping overnight.
report card	5. Good boy—you got 3 As this time.
Florida	6. We went to Disney World® last summer.
help	7. Will you buy some Girl Scout cookies?
ouch!	8. I got a sliver in my thumb.
lost	9. Where is my jacket?
carpool	10. It's my mother's turn to drive today.

6.1.18. Clue Words: Colloquial Sentences

repair	1. Do you know how to fix a flat tire on your bicycle?
boots	2. I bought some boots yesterday.
temperature	3. The paper said it would be much warmer tomorrow.
mail	4. I like to get letters and post cards.
rest	5. How many hours do you sleep at night?
mistake	6. Do you have an eraser?
doormat	7. Wipe the mud off your shoes before you come into the house.
store	8. Will you please stop for the groceries on your way home from school?
capital	9. Where does the governor live?
tingles	10. I hit my elbow on the corner of my desk.

6.1.19. Clue Words: Colloquial Sentences

resort	1. Have you ever been to a dude ranch?
game	2. Our family likes to go bowling.

bashful	3. My little sister is very shy in front of strangers.
magic	4. Do you know how to do any card tricks?
vitamin C	5. We always have orange juice for breakfast.
dull	6. These scissors are not sharp enough to cut paper.
startled	7. The car back-fired and made me jump.
hobby	8. I would like to be a spelunker and explore caves.
snack	9. I brought an apple to eat at recess.
kites	10. The boys are flying kites in the vacant lot.
cold	11. It snowed last night and the ground is frozen.
60¢	12. How much do you have to pay for a double ice cream cone?

6.1.20. Clue Words: Colloquial Sentences

siren	1. The fire engine made so much noise I covered my ears.
safety	2. We have good brakes on our car.
party	3. We had ice cream and cake at the birthday party.
holiday	4. Halloween is the time for tricks or treats and fun.
afraid	5. Our cat ran under the porch when it saw a mouse.
parakeet	6. My parakeet says, "Well, hello there," when anyone comes into our house.
toy	7. I have an electric train that my father likes to play with.
February	8. Can you name four holidays that are observed in this month?
buffalo	9. What is the difference between a buffalo and a bison? (none)
sport	10. Baseball is my favorite game and I like (team) best.

*6.1.21. Clue Words: Colloquial Sentences**

eating	1. We went to McDonald's last night for dinner.
circus	2. The circus will be here next week and my brother is taking me.
family	3. Do you have any brothers or sisters?
accident	4. I fell off my skateboard and hurt my knee.
baking	5. My mother just made a batch of chocolate chip cookies.
taste	6. They have a new flavor at the ice cream shop.
measurement	7. How tall are you without your shoes?
bakery	8. She ate three doughnuts at the store.
shopping	9. I got a new pair of shoes for school.
playground	10. Let's play volleyball after school.

6.2. BEGINNING ADULTS

6.2.1. Clue Words: Colloquial Sentences

caution	
look & listen	1. Be careful not to fall on those steep steps.
look	2. The steps are slippery.
listen	3. It has been raining.
exercise	
look & listen	1. Do you exercise every day?
look	2. I walk three miles every day.
listen	3. Sometimes I jog.
weather	
look & listen	1. This is a beautiful day.
look	2. There is not a cloud in the sky.
listen	3. It has been warm all day.
food	
look & listen	1. What do you eat for breakfast?
look	2. I like a big breakfast.
listen	3. Breakfast is my favorite meal.
telephone	
look & listen	1. Can you hear on the telephone?

*Contributed by Nancy Bettenhausen.

	look	2. What is your telephone number?
	listen	3. Call me sometime.
recreation		
	look & listen	1. Golf is my favorite game.
	look	2. Do you play golf?
	listen	3. A very popular game is ______.
parade		
	look & listen	1. Do you watch the Rose Parade on TV?
	look	2. It is a beautiful sight.
	listen	3. I love a parade.
speed		
	look & listen	1. He drives his car too fast.
	look	2. Last week he got a ticket.
	listen	3. What is the speed limit?

6.2.2. Clue Words: Colloquial Sentences

radio		
	look & listen	1. I like to hear the news every morning over ______.
	look	2. I always listen for the weather report.
	listen	3. Oh dear, more rain.
crowds		
	look & listen	1. There were hundreds of people at the beaches over the weekend.
	look	2. We were some of the crowd.
	listen	3. We all got a sunburn.
gusty		
	look & listen	1. There were strong winds from the north last week.
	look	2. Cold weather will soon be here.
	listen	3. Winter is on the way.
hash		
	look & listen	1. We had roast beef for dinner yesterday.
	look	2. Today we had roast lamb.
	listen	3. What do you do with leftovers?
memory		
	look & listen	1. She says she never forgets a face.

	look	2. But she has trouble remembering names.
	listen	3. That's my problem too.
fun		
	look & listen	1. We are having a barbeque next weekend.
	look	2. Bring your whole family.
	listen	3. The more the merrier!
fishing		
	look & listen	1. We are going fishing next week.
	look	2. The boat leaves the pier at four in the morning.
	listen	3. I hope I won't be seasick.

*6.2.3. Clue Words: Colloquial Sentences**

expensive	1. Most vacations cost more than you plan.
	2. Food costs more than lodging.
	3. Next time we will economize and camp.
confused	1. She drove the wrong way on the boulevard.
	2. She did not see the traffic sign.
	3. Lucky for her no citation.
tired	1. I can't climb any more stairs.
	2. This apartment should have an elevator.
	3. The walk up three flights is exhausting.
game	1. Do you know how to play chess?
	2. Yes. Shall we play a game?
	3. I'll have to learn first.
encourage	1. If I practice I know I can learn to do it.
	2. Practice makes perfect they say.
	3. Speechread more and you will improve.
rush	1. The cars go by here too fast.
	2. I'm sure they exceed the speed limit.
	3. What is the speed limit in the city?
distance	1. Is it too far to walk to town?
	2. It's about four miles from here.
	3. That's too far for me.
prepare	1. What time shall we start fixing dinner?
	2. Friends are coming tonight about seven.
	3. Will you make the salad?

*Contributed by Gayle Bishop and adapted.

6.2.4. Clue Words: Colloquial Sentences

vacation	1. We plan to go east next summer.
	2. We have friends in Chicago.
	3. What is the capital of Illinois?
camping	1. Do you like to go camping?
	2. Have you ever slept out under the stars?
	3. I prefer a tent overhead!
furniture	1. Her home is filled with beautiful old furniture.
	2. Most of it belonged to her family.
	3. I like the Danish modern style.
stories	1. Did you read fairy tales as a child?
	2. What was your favorite story?
	3. Remember Aesop's fables?
beverage	1. Will you have cream and sugar in your coffee?
	2. Coffee keeps me awake.
	3. So does tea!
home	1. We plan to build a house next year.
	2. It will be a ranch style house.
	3. And it will be all on one floor.
gem	1. What is your birthstone?
	2. The birthstone for April is a diamond.
	3. Diamonds are a girl's best friend.

6.2.5. Clue Words: Colloquial Sentences

dessert	1. Apple pie is the favorite American dessert.
	2. Do you prefer pie, ice cream, or cake for dessert?
	3. My favorite is any pie a la mode.
13	1. Are you superstitious?
	2. Some will not walk under a ladder.
	3. How do you feel about a black cat?
wish	1. Have you ever wished upon a star?
	2. Do you remember—star light, star bright?
	3. Can you say all the rhyme?
movie	1. There is a good movie on TV tonight.

	2. I like to watch old westerns.
	3. Who is your favorite movie star?
weekend	1. We are going to spend the weekend with friends at the beach.
	2. This weekend will be a vacation.
	3. It is a three-day holiday.
exercise	1. He walks three miles to work every morning.
	2. It takes him about an hour to get to the office.
	3. I would be exhausted!
job	1. I am looking for a job.
	2. A part time job would be ok.
	3. Four hours a day is all I want.

*6.2.6. Clue Words: Colloquial Sentences**

time	1. It's getting late.
catalogue	2. I will order the merchandise by mail.
detergents	3. I must buy laundry soap when I go to the store.
recollect	4. Can't you remember who telephoned?
siblings	5. She had three brothers and two sisters.
protection	6. Do you wear sunglasses?
engaged	7. What a lovely diamond ring.
weather	8. It is a warm and sunny morning.
sensation	9. My palm has been itching for two days.
broke	10. I bought four pairs of shoes (boots) that I really didn't need and now I'm short until pay day.
manicure	11. I file and polish my fingernails at least once a week.
money	12. It costs senior citizens only a dime to take a bus downtown.
store	13. Did you do your food shopping for the week?
oops!	14. I spilled coffee all over my new coat.

*Contributed by Melody Stouffer and Gloria Feld.

*6.2.7. Clue Words: Colloquial Sentences**

Clue Words	Colloquial Sentences
expensive	1. I went to the store today and prices are outrageous.
raise	2. After you're with the company for six months, your salary will be increased.
fear	3. I dread going to the dentist.
tired	4. I had a rough day at work.
climate	5. The weather is so unpredictable.
eating	6. Let's go out for dinner tomorrow.
illness	7. I had the Hong Kong flu for two weeks.
problems	8. Everything went haywire today.
broke	9. Can you lend me ten bucks until next pay day?
hearing aid	10. How long do your batteries last?

6.2.8. Clue Words: Colloquial Sentences

Clue Words	Colloquial Sentences
time	1. It takes me forty-five minutes to walk home from class.
advice	2. Do you ever drive from the back seat of your car?
fine	3. Have you ever had a ticket for speeding?
likeness	4. Is the picture on your driver's license a good one?
busy	5. I have a thousand things to do today!
seafood	6. He is very fond of oysters on the half shell.
superior	7. That was the best pie I ever ate.
early	8. He always gets to class ahead of time.
boss	9. That teacher of ours is a slave-driver.
secret	10. Please don't breathe a word of this to anyone.
expensive	11. We didn't buy the house because the price was too high.
evaluate	12. You can't judge people by their looks.

6.2.9. Clue Words: Colloquial Sentences

Clue Words	Colloquial Sentences
annoy	1. Children like to tease each other.

*Contributed by Maxine Orlikoff.

mistake	2. She found an error in her bank balance.
clever	3. The boy has a keen mind and is a good student.
decline	4. I am sorry I will be unable to accept your invitation to lunch.
inactive	5. We spent a lazy weekend at home.
tidy	6. Her house is always orderly and neat.
wealthy	7. The family has become affluent with investments in real estate.
ticket	8. We had to pay a fine for speeding on the freeway.
landslide	9. The election was an overwhelming victory for the candidate.
played out	10. She says she works so hard to lipread that she is exhausted after class.
skillful	11. He is a most competent surgeon.
document	12. Do we get a diploma when this term is over?

6.2.10. Clue Words: Colloquial Sentences

flowers	1. My garden should be beautiful this year.
newspaper	2. More people buy the Sunday edition of the paper than the daily issues.
home	3. Our friends bought a trailer and are living in Florida this winter.
telephone	4. I would call you oftener but every time I try to reach you the line is busy.
styles	5. What do you think the fashion will be for skirt lengths this fall?
spring	6. The fruit trees are in full bloom.
fib	7. Have you ever told a little white lie?
forgot	8. I left my umbrella on the bus.
pill	9. Don't forget to take your vitamins.
exercise	10. How far can you run without getting out of breath?
chilly	11. It is cold enough for a fire in the fireplace.
money	12. How much are the new cars?

6.2.11. Clue Words: Colloquial Sentences

erudite	1.	She speaks seven languages fluently.
dessert	2.	Do you know where I can buy some good chocolate eclairs?
golf	3.	Is your average game under par?
poison	4.	Be sure to keep medicine out of the reach of children.
callow	5.	The boy was immature for his age.
imperative	6.	He felt it was necessary to make the trip to Washington.
articulate	7.	She expresses herself very well.
sultry	8.	The weather has been very humid lately.
tact	9.	She is not fat, just pleasingly plump!
odor	10.	Someone is cooking onions.
idea	11.	I just had a brainstorm—let's stop for coffee.
day-dream	12.	That boy always seems to have his head in the clouds.

6.2.12. Clue Words: Colloquial Sentences

bargain	1.	I bought three pairs of shoes at the sale.
recreation	2.	He plays golf every day.
exercise	3.	I took a long walk this morning.
trip	4.	Where did you go over the weekend?
draft	5.	Will you please shut the window—I feel a cold wind.
meat	6.	I bought a leg of lamb for Sunday dinner.
shopping	7.	I like to buy my groceries on Thursday.
house	8.	We have our home up for sale.
pie	9.	What is your favorite dessert?
autumn	10.	The leaves are beginning to change color.
veterinarian	11.	We had to take the dog to the doctor for rabies shots.
lost	12.	Where did I put my car keys?
healthful	13.	Do you believe an apple a day keeps the doctor away?
cook	14.	She makes the best pies.

6.2.13. Clue Words: Colloquial Sentences

surf	1. We watched the huge waves pound on the shore.
draft	2. Is the breeze from the window too cold for you?
leisure	3. We had the day off and went to lunch and a movie.
recreation	4. Shall we bowl for an hour before lunch?
sun	5. The bright light made my eyes water.
heirloom	6. The old pewter tea pot belonged to my grandmother.
gift	7. She brought me some flowers from her garden.
jaywalking	8. How large a fine did you have to pay?
crowd	9. Thousands of people watched the parade.
choice	10. We would like to have you come for dinner either Friday or Saturday evening.
speechless	11. I was scared to death!
How's that again?	12. What? (did you say)

*6.2.14. Clue Words: Colloquial Sentences**

warning	1. I told him to be more careful.
flowers	2. Asters are beautiful, but I prefer chrysanthemums.
telephone	3. I called three times but there was no answer.
hospital	4. I'm sorry, she can't have visitors today.
weekend	5. What are your plans for Saturday and Sunday?
afraid?	6. I want to get home before dark.
coins	7. Don't forget to take some money for the parking meter.
talented	8. She plays the piano and sings very well.
food	9. She served chicken salad, muffins, and blueberry pie for lunch.
recall	10. How well can you remember what was just said?

*Contributed by Peggy Sandford and adapted.

ambidextrous	11. He can write with either hand.
tough?	12. His bark is worse than his bite.

6.2.15. Clue Words: Colloquial Sentences

chilly	1. I think I will get my sweater. There is a cold wind blowing.
agree	2. My opinion is the same as yours.
surf	3. An eight-foot wave struck the boat.
flowers	4. Her garden is lovely at this time of the year.
give up	5. The doctor told him he should stop smoking.
sorry	6. It is a shame you had to miss the concert.
relative	7. She is my father's sister.
lazy	8. I don't feel much like working today.
summer	9. It's so crowded on the beach you can't find a place to sit down.
pie	10. Will you help me to peel the apples while I make the crust?
excuse me	11. I'm sorry, I didn't mean to interrupt what you were saying.
hair style	12. Men don't have to go to the barber as often these days with longer hair the vogue.

6.2.16. Clue Words: Colloquial Sentences

letter	1. Be sure to write while you are away.
Monday	2. For some reason we always wash clothes on the same day.
polishing	3. He is washing and waxing his new car.
sport	4. She is a baseball fan.
telephone	5. I'll call you tonight after seven o'clock.
misplaced	6. I can't seem to find my house key.
outing	7. We went on an all-day picnic last Saturday.
hobby	8. Photography is called the number one hobby in the United States.
library	9. I have to return some books today.
fortune	10. She said she is waiting for her ship to come in.

bridge	11. Have you ever bid a grand slam?
relax	12. You can rest better with your feet on a footstool.
reading	13. I sat up half the night to finish that exciting book.
jaywalking	14. Don't cross the street in the middle of the block.
speech	15. Slang expressions often become accepted idiom in our language.

6.2.17. Clue Words: Colloquial Sentences

Note to teacher: For the following sentences a choice of either clue words, underlined words to indicate use of more voice, or both procedures are suggested.

memory	1. Did you remember to bring a pencil?
noise	2. The people next door keep their television on all day.
hurry?	3. You seem to be in a rush this morning.
weekend	4. Did you go to ________ for Saturday and Sunday?
visit	5. We spent a short time with friends from out of town.
hedge	6. Our neighbors planted (oleander, lilacs, etc.) across the back of their property.
author	7. Do you know who wrote the continued story in the *Ladies Home Journal?*
material	8. What kind of cloth is in that suit?
late	9. I thought you were never coming.
non-stop	10. We flew directly from here to (Miami, Chicago, etc.).
practice	11. Do you try to do some speechreading every day?
change	12. Tomorrow I am going to paint the fence white.

*6.2.18. Clue Words: Colloquial Sentences**

Clue Words	Colloquial Sentences
newspaper	1. Our paper boy always seems to throw the paper into the shrubbery.
movie	2. We seldom see a movie until it comes to our local theater.
advertising	3. Don't you simply hate all those silly commercials on television?
music	4. We went to the (music center, auditorium) and heard a wonderful Beethoven concert.
traffic	5. There was a terrible jam on the freeway this morning.
reading	6. Have you spent much time in the library this semester?
groceries	7. We went to the market yesterday and bought a week's supply of food.
vacation	8. Would you rather go to the mountains or to the seashore next summer?
weather	9. We haven't had very many warm, sunny days this winter.
friendly	10. They always seem so happy to have people stop by at any time.

6.2.19. Clue Words: Colloquial Sentences

Clue Words	Colloquial Sentences
caution	1. Be careful not to fall on these steep stairs.
advice	2. My grandfather said if you want good exercise try sawing wood.
weather	3. It's awfully raw and windy today.
wharf	4. We are going down to the pier to try the fishing.
teacher	5. She has a large class of third graders this year.
food tradition	6. Do you like cranberry sauce with your turkey?
transportation	7. I think I will get a new car in the spring.
recreation	8. Would you care to play eighteen holes of golf on Saturday?

*Contributed by Ruth Reed.

fall	9. Now is the time to cut back the roses.
expense	10. I made a long distance call to my friend but we only had a short talk.
remember	11. Don't forget to vote (next week).
breakfast	12. How will you have your eggs—boiled, fried, or scrambled?
overtime	13. He decided to stay at the office and plow through all the work.
Clairol®	14. Her hair used to be brown; I didn't recognize her as a blonde.
smile	15. Wipe that frown off your face and try to look cheerful.

Chapter 7

SIMPLE STORIES

Elementary Stories Presented in a Series of Closely Related Sentences

SIMPLE STORIES follow colloquial sentences cued by clue words in Beginning Speechreading instruction. The word "simple" is not meant to imply that the content presented is mediocre and without interest. The simple story consists of a series of closely related sentences which follow in logical sequence. The subject matter is highly familiar in content for both children and adults. This kind of exercise may be enhanced with a humorous punch line or ending. Examples of these stories are *A Mouse in My House* for children and *The English Teacher* for adults found in the following section.

Care should be taken to reword a story for visibility if a familiar tale or fable is given. In most of these stories the outcome is predictable. Restatement and redundancy are helpful adjuncts to the simple story. The sentences should be short and highly visible, and in addition, familiar vocabulary should be used.

To present a simple story the title is written on the board. The teacher then gives each sentence using a reduced voice with pupils responding to every sentence. It is *important* that the instructor repeats the student responses to insure all students understand. After completing the story the teacher may say: "Now close your eyes and think about the story. I will retell some of the important parts. Tell me what you hear." Using more voice she gives the highlights while students listen only. For any pupil with a loss severe enough to miss the audible retelling, the teacher needs to reassure that person to watch and speechread. A student volunteer may give the story to the class.

7.1. SIMPLE STORIES FOR CHILDREN

These stories are arranged in approximate order of difficulty with relation to vocabulary and concepts for children.

7.1.1. Body Parts—Something to do at the Chalkboard

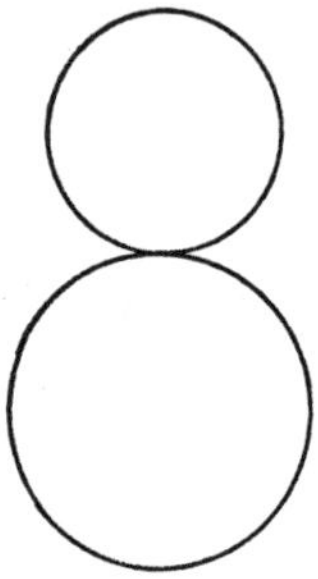

Figure 6.

PROCEDURE: Two circles are drawn on the board preceding the lesson. The teacher, with reduced voice, begins the exercise. Volunteers may add to the picture as the teacher gives the information. Each child may draw his own picture at the same time.

What is this? This is a boy. The poor boy! He doesn't have any arms. Who can give him some arms? The boy should have hands. Now the boy has a head, a body, two arms, and two hands. He needs legs. Let's make him a tall boy. Make his legs long. Give the boy two feet. Is this all the boy needs? Of course he must have eyes to see. He must have ears to hear. He must have a mouth to smile. Don't forget his nose. He wants to smell the food mother is cooking. Put some hair on his head. Now give him a name. Look at him carefully. Can you think of anything more to put on the boy? (eyebrows, eyelashes, toes, fingers, fingernails, feet, etc.) What name did you give him?

Variation: Dress the boy for a second lesson.

7.1.2. Our Family

What is a family? I don't know, but my mother is part of our family. My father is part of our family. My brother is part of our family. My sister is part of our family. My grandmother belongs to our family. My uncle is part of our family. My aunt belongs to our family. My cousins belong to our family. I guess almost everybody belongs to our family. Who belongs to yours?

*7.1.3. The Big Balloon**

My balloon is red. It is a big balloon. I bounce my balloon. I fly my balloon. My balloon is fun. It came from the fair. It is filled with special stuff. The stuff makes the balloon magic. My balloon won't break. It won't go pop. It will last and last. Would you like to share my balloon with me?

7.1.4. The New Baby†

We have a new baby at our house. It is a boy. His name is Robert. But we call him Bobby. Bobby is a big baby. He is only three weeks old but he weighs 12 pounds. The doctor says he is a very healthy baby. Bobby has blue eyes. He hasn't any hair — just fuzz. My mother thinks he has a beautifully shaped head. She says he will be a smart man. She said he might be President of the United States someday. He sleeps most of the time. But he cries when he is hungry. Sometimes my mother lets me feed him. I hold the bottle while he drinks. This is fun. He squints his eyes at me. I think he is trying to laugh at me. I hope he grows fast so I can play with him. If he gets to be President of the United States I will go visit him in Washington.

7.1.5. Watching Airplanes

One day my father took me to the airport. We watched the airplanes take off. We watched them come in. When they came down they made a lot of noise. When they took off I had to put my hands over my ears. My father said, "Watch the airplane fly away." It got smaller and smaller. I wanted to have a ride in an airplane. So one day we got on a plane. We went so fast. When we were way up in the air I said, "When are we going to get smaller and smaller?" My father laughed and laughed.

7.1.6. My Puppy

I have a puppy. He is only three months old. I got him for my birthday. We play together. He likes to play ball. When I

*Contributed by Joan Kolodin.
†Contributed by Alta Taylor.

throw the ball he runs fast. He tries to catch the ball. Then he brings it back to me. His name is ______. I will teach him tricks. I will teach him how to roll over. I gave him a bone to chew on. The bone makes his teeth strong. His teeth are really strong. Yesterday he tore my shirt. My mother was mad at ______.

7.1.7. You Know What?

Tomorrow is my birthday. I am going to have a party. And you know what? I will be 5 years old. My mother said I could invite 5 of my friends. And you know what? We are going to have ice cream and a birthday cake. We will play games. And you know what? I can hardly wait. I wish it was tomorrow. Then it would be my birthday.

*7.1.8. The Zoo**

Last Saturday we went to the zoo. We went to see all the animals. The first animal we saw was the elephant. He was big and had a very long trunk. He reached his trunk out for some peanuts. And he put them in his mouth. Then, he wanted more. But we did not have any more, so we said good-bye. Then we went to see the lion. He was big and mean and he looked hungry. When he growled we were frightened and we ran away. When we stopped running we were hungry too. We saw a hot dog stand and we all had two hot dogs. All of a sudden we heard a lot of noise. People were running toward the monkey cage. So we started running to see what was happening. There was a monkey eating a banana. And a little monkey was throwing water at him. The big monkey got mad. And he chased the little monkey all around the cage. After watching all that running and chasing, we were tired. And we went home.

*7.1.9. Shopping**

I like to go shopping with my mother. We went downtown shopping last Saturday. I wanted a new dress. I tried on four

---

Contributed by Mary Martin.

*Contributed by Marilyn Lonsbury and adapted.

dresses. One was a pretty blue dress. I said, "This is the one I want." My mother liked it too. She bought the dress for me. Then we looked for shoes. We found some blue shoes that matched the dress. Mother bought the shoes and then we went to lunch. After lunch we stopped at a candy store. We bought some of our favorite candy. Do you know what kind that is? — peanut brittle. Then we went home. We were tired, but it was fun. I think I had more fun than my mother.

7.1.10. *Fourth of July Parade*†

Bob is a Boy Scout. His Boy Scout troop loves to march. They were invited to march in the 4th of July Parade. Bob was happy. Bob polished his shoes. Bob polished the buckle of his belt. Bob pressed his pants and shirt and scarf. Bob put these things on and joined the troop. The parade began. The boy Scouts marched. They marched and marched some more. They marched farther and farther. Bob's feet were tired. Bob's face was warm. When would the parade be over? Finally they reached the judges. The judges said, "First prize to the Boy Scout troop." Was it worth it? Bob thought, "I suppose so. But I think I'll sit and watch the parade next year."

7.1.11. *Jim's Question: Why Do Dogs Chase Rabbits?**

One day Jim and I were hunting. Jim is five years old. We saw a rabbit. Our dog saw the rabbit too. He began to chase the rabbit. Jim asked me, "Why do dogs chase rabbits?" This is how I answered Jim's question. Do you like to play baseball? Or run in an open field? Or swing on a swing? Or blow a whistle? Or beat a drum? Do you like to wave at a train? Do you like to run until you are out of breath? These are things most children like to do. There are things that animals like to do too. A cat likes to warm itself in the sun. It likes to wash its face. It cleans itself with its tongue. A dog likes to bury bones. It likes to bark. It likes to wag its tail. When he sees a rabbit, he wants to run after it. He races the rabbit to its hole. The rabbit usually wins. But it was a fine race, wasn't it?

---

†Contributed by Joan Kolodin.

*Contributed by John Cavanagh.

*7.1.12. Whiskers**

I had a rabbit. His name was Whiskers. He had long, long hairs from his nose that looked like whiskers. Whiskers was very smart. He was also very strong. He slept in a big box that used to have a piano in it. It was a very big box. Whiskers loved to run and play. One morning I woke up to find he had disappeared. I couldn't find him in his box. I couldn't find him in the yard. I couldn't find him anywhere. Finally, a neighbor called to say a rabbit was sitting under a bush. I ran over to her house and sure enough, there was Whiskers. He was winking up at me from under the bush. He was saying, "Fooled you, didn't I!" I grabbed him and took him home. When I got home, I put him in his box. Whiskers ran to a corner of it. I looked very hard and what do you think I found? There in the corner was a little hole. It was just big enough for a rabbit to squeeze through. Whiskers hadn't disappeared. He had gone out his own back door.

7.1.13. Guess What I Saw (or Man From Outer Space)†

One day I saw a little man. He was a funny little man. He was all green. First I looked at his face. Then I looked at his forehead. Can you guess what I saw? I saw two small horns. They were growing right out of the top of his forehead. I said, "Little man, where did you come from?" "I came from outer space," said the little green man. Then he pointed his finger to a tree. I went to the tree. Under the tree was a strange thing. It was a space ship. I looked in the space ship. It looked like a little baby house with a steering wheel. Ho, ho, ho! What a funny space ship. Ho, ho, ho! What a funny little green man. I looked – where was the little green man. I looked up. I looked down. I looked all around. Then bump! Something hit me. I looked up. The little green man was in the tree. He threw an apple at me. Bump! He said, "Ho, ho, ho! I think you are funny too." Down he came. He jumped into the space ship. Away he flew. Oh, dear! Mother will never believe me!

---

*Contributed by Nancy Bettenhausen.
†Contributed by Shirley Nelin.

7.2. BEGINNING ADULTS

*7.2.1. Softball, Anyone?**

My daughter Dawn belongs to a softball team. The softball team plays ball on Sunday. The team needs all the cheering they can get. The whole family goes out to give the team some moral support. My youngest daughter, Tracie, likes to cheer for her sister. One Sunday, Tracie was the star of the game. She caught the softball. She did not catch the ball with a glove. She caught the ball right in the eye! Two hours later her eye was very swollen. Then it turned black and blue. It was quite a shiner! The next Sunday, Tracie said that she did not want to go to the game. I could not understand why. Her sister could not understand why. Can you?

7.2.2. A Fishing Trip

Last week my father, brother, and I (our family) went fishing. We got up early in the morning. It was long before sunrise. We had to drive about 75 miles to the lake. We got there just as the sun was coming up. The weather was beautiful. We bought some bait and rented a boat. It was an old rowboat with a motor on the back. About one-half mile out on the lake the motor stopped. "Where is all the water in the bottom of the boat coming from?" I asked. "It is nothing to be worried about," said my father. "Here is a pail — you bail out a little water. I'll row the boat." We finally dropped anchor, but I kept on bailing. "Don't you want to fish?" said my father. "No, thanks, I'd rather be sure to stay afloat," was my answer. The men fished and fished. I bailed and bailed. At last they had their limit of fish. We started for the shore. "The fishing was great," said the men. "Let's come again next week." I'm going to stay home.

7.2.3. Our New Car

We have a new car. We bought it last week. We shopped a long time before we bought it. Everyone in the family wanted a different car. The boys wanted a car with power and speed. I

*Contributed by May Laughlin.

don't like to go too fast. The girls wanted an expensive convertible. The convertibles use too much gas. We looked at compacts. They were not too expensive. The gas mileage was good. The salesman said we could get 30 miles to a gallon of gas. But our family cannot get into a compact car at one time. The boys want room for their long legs. I do not like to be crowded. We looked at large cars. They are too hard to park. We finally looked at a medium sized car. It was the right price. Do you want to know what we bought? I drove it today. Come on outside and I'll take you for a ride.

*7.2.4. An English Lesson**

This is the story about a young woman. She was teaching a class in English. One day she was teaching the proper use of *I* after *It is.* Many of her students were making the same mistake. They would say, "It is me." She wrote examples on the board. Then she wrote all over the board "It is I — It is I — It is I." She was writing in the corner next to the door. Suddenly the door opened and she was bumped. The person who opened the door was the principal. He was startled and said "Who did I bump?" And what did she say? "Oh! It's me, the teacher." Then she said to her class, "What was just said in this room that was incorrect?" A boy raised his hand and said, "I know, teacher." She said, "What was it?" He answered, "The principal should have said "Whom did I bump?"

*7.2.5. The Science Experiment**

Susie bought some plants. They were flowers. She put some flowers in one room. These flowers heard fine music many days. She put some flowers in another room. These flowers heard much noise and rock music many days. The flowers received the same water. The flowers received the same sunshine. Only the music was not the same. Can you guess what happened? Yes! You are right. The flowers that heard fine music got bigger and bigger. The flowers that heard noise and rock music began to wilt. The

---

*Contributed by Anne Gabriels.

*Contributed by Joan Kolodin.

science teacher was pleased with Susie's experiment. The experiment was a success. But Susie was sad. She was sad because she likes rock music.

7.2.6. *Eating at the Movies**

Do you like to go to the movies? When I go I like to eat popcorn and drink soda pop. Usually, I share the popcorn and soda pop with my husband. We also have a habit of being late. It's very hard to find a seat in the theater after the movie starts. It's so dark and your eyes just cannot focus fast enough. One night we were late as usual, and we had popcorn and soda pop as usual. We found a seat and I was just starting to focus my eyes. I saw from the corner of my eyes that the popcorn cup my husband was holding was already half empty. I thought I had better get some before it was all gone. I reached over quickly and my fingers dived in. Oh, was that cold! and wet! It was not popcorn I felt — but icy cold soda pop — all the way up to my knuckles. In the dark, the popcorn cup and the soda pop cup looked the same. They certainly don't feel the same.

7.2.7. *My Remodeled Kitchen*†

We have just remodeled our kitchen. First we painted the walls. We kept our old sink, but we put new tiles around it. We threw out the old stove. We bought a new built-in stove. Our refrigerator was very old. We bought a big refrigerator-freezer. It matches the stove. The refrigerator holds three times more food than the old one did. The freezer holds 100 pounds of food. We had our wood cabinets stained dark brown. They look really sharp! They blend in with the new stove and refrigerator. We also bought a dishwasher. No more dishpan hands.

7.2.8. *My Dog***

My dog is just like one of our family. He has a bed he sleeps in just like we do. He eats breakfast at the same time we eat

*Contributed by Nancy Bettenhausen.
†Contributed by Lois Fraud and adapted.
**Contributed by Russell Harvey.

ours. Then he goes outside to play. He loves to run and chase birds and insects (bugs). Sometimes I throw a ball and then try to catch him. He runs so fast I hardly ever catch him. When he is tired he takes a nap. Sometimes in the afternoon we take him for a walk. We take him for a ride in the car. He gets his hair cut and has a bath once a month. His life would look like fun to many people. Do you ever wish you led a dog's life?

7.2.9. Cold Feet and Socks†

I decided to go camping. I had never been camping before. I went camping with my brother. We went to Yosemite. There was snow on the ground at Yosemite. A beautiful white blanket of snow. The snow was cold. The air was cold. And I was very cold. I wore three pairs of socks the first night. The next morning, when I woke up, my feet were extremely cold. I couldn't wiggle (move) my toes. I warmed my feet in some warm water. Oh, did that feel good! The second night I wore four pairs of socks to bed. Again I woke up with cold, cold feet. On the third night, I wore five pairs of socks. I wore knee socks, thermal socks, and fuzzy socks. But even with five pairs of socks, my feet were still cold. Guess how many pairs of socks I wore on the fourth night? I wore six pairs of socks. And still my feet were numb from the cold. We cut our trip short. We came home a day earlier than we planned. I ran out of socks to wear.

*7.2.10. My First Airplane Ride**

I took my first airplane trip to Arizona. I was scared for two days before the trip. My mother told me not to be frightened – it would be fun. The day came and she made me a big breakfast. That was a mistake. By the time I got to the airport my stomach hurt. The plane did not leave on time. Take-off was delayed an hour. This made me more nervous. We finally took off. The captain's voice came over the intercom. He said, "Good morning, ladies and gentlemen. Welcome to Flight 432, Los Angeles to Phoenix. Please keep your seat belt fastened. We will

†Contributed by Maxene Orlikoff.

*Contributed by Sherri Shiroshi and adapted.

encounter some turbulence for a short time." Oh me! I was feeling worse by the minute. The plane went up and down. My stomach went down and up. Just then the stewardess said, "Would you like some coffee?" I shut my eyes and said, "No thank you." As we approached Arizona the woman sitting next to me pointed out the desert below us. I couldn't even turn my head to look out the window. Finally we landed. Was that a relief. But now I had to think about the trip back. Coming home the ride was even more rough. Next time I'll take the bus. Flying is for the birds!

Chapter 8

TOPIC SENTENCES

Advanced Speechreading Material

TOPIC SENTENCES PROVIDE a stimulating challenge to the advanced speechreader. The sentences are often longer and contain information of a broader context. The method of presentation is similar to that of colloquial sentences clued by words, except as just stated the language is less familiar, conveys more information, and is usually not understood at the first reading. For this reason the topic sentence must be expanded for comprehension by the use of clue sentences.

This is the kind of statement that might be heard in a situation where people are exchanging ideas without being aware the hard-of-hearing need supportive information to understand what was said. How does the topic sentence procedure assist the hard-of-hearing follow ideas which are elaborately stated? By giving the hearing-impaired clue sentences which support the topic sentence, he is auding and speechreading the "bits and pieces" to make an integrated whole and reach a perceptual closure.

PROCEDURE: The instructor writes a clue word or words on the board establishing the topic. The sentence is then read. The teacher asks if anyone knows the gist of it. Before a restatement of the topic sentence is given, clue sentences are introduced which help establish the vocabulary and provide those who missed the first reading with needed information. These sentences are repeated by class members who volunteer the information. The topic sentence is then repeated. A pupil gives the essence of the statement. An example follows.

Clue Words: Legal Adults

Topic Sentence: Most of our fifty states have dropped the age of legal adulthood from the traditional age of twenty-one to eighteen or nineteen so that today young citizens can vote, serve on juries, and make contracts.

Clue Sentences:

1. There are fifty United States.
2. Twenty-one years was the legal age for adulthood.
3. Many states have changed their laws.
4. What is the legal voting age in our state?

Return to the original topic sentence.

This same technique may be reversed for intermediate students. The clue word and clue sentences are given before the topic sentence. The clue sentences must have greater elaboration with attention paid to visible language. Give the clue sentences with some voice. Then the topic sentence is presented with greatly reduced voice. When sentences are presented at this level the teacher might use the Listen only procedure for the topic sentence.

8.1. TOPIC SENTENCES

8.1.1. Clue Word: Redwood Tree

Topic Sentence: The tallest living thing in the world is a redwood tree in northern California.

Clue Sentences:

1. Redwood trees are very tall.
2. Where are redwood trees found?
3. How tall are they said to be?

8.1.2. Clue Words: The White House

Topic Sentence: The White House got its name from the white paint used to cover the damage caused by fire during the War of 1812.

Clue Sentences:

1. Our house should have a new coat of paint.

2. Paint can cover damage caused by a fire.
3. What happened to the White House in 1812?

8.1.3. Clue Word: Air Mail

TOPIC SENTENCE: The carriage of air mail, inaugurated by the United States Government in 1918, was the foundation for all commercial aviation in this country.

CLUE SENTENCES:

1. Most mail goes by air today.
2. When did the United States Government start air mail?
3. Commercial aviation began soon after air mail was inaugurated.

Repeat the original sentence.

8.1.4. Clue Word: Chalk

TOPIC SENTENCE: The chalk we use when we write at the board in school is a very soft powdery limestone composed chiefly of fossil shells of tiny animals that once lived in the sea.

CLUE SENTENCES:

1. Chalk is very soft and powdery.
2. Chalk is limestone.
3. Limestone is made up of fossil sea shells.
4. Tiny animals once lived in these sea shells.

8.1.5. Clue Words: Flag Day

TOPIC SENTENCE: Flag Day commemorates the adoption of the Stars and Stripes by the Continental Congress, but not until 1949 did it become a national Flag Day.

CLUE SENTENCES:

1. We celebrate a holiday in June.
2. June 14th is Flag Day.
3. When did Flag Day become a national observance?

8.1.6. Clue Words: New Year's Day

TOPIC SENTENCE: New Year's Day had its origin in Roman times when sacrifices were made to the two-faced god Janus, who looked back on the past and forward to the future.

CLUE SENTENCES:

1. We celebrate New Year's Day on January first.
2. This is a very old celebration.
3. Who were the first people to observe New Year's Day?
4. The month of January was named for a Roman god.

8.1.7. Clue Word: Easter

TOPIC SENTENCE: Easter is on a different date each year because it must fall on a Sunday; it must be after the full moon; and it must be on or after the first day of Spring.

CLUE SENTENCES:

1. Do you know how to figure out when Easter will occur each year?
2. First you must know the date of the full moon.
3. Next you must know the date of the first day of Spring.
4. Then you must know the date of the first Sunday after the full moon that is after the first day of Spring.

8.1.8. Clue Word: Lincoln Penny

TOPIC SENTENCE: Have you ever looked closely at a Lincoln penny on the side opposite the head and observed the Lincoln Memorial and the very tiny statue inside it?

CLUE SENTENCES:

1. Do you have a penny in your pocket or purse?
2. On one side is the head of Abraham Lincoln.
3. What is on the other side of the penny?
4. Look at it carefully.
5. Can you see a very small statue?

8.1.9. Clue Word: Blinking

TOPIC SENTENCE: Did you know the fastest automatic action of the body is blinking the eyelids, which spreads moisture over the eyeball and takes only 1/20th of a second?

CLUE SENTENCES:

1. Wink your eye!

2. That action does not take very long.
3. Blinking the eye is an automatic action.
4. It takes only a fraction of a second to do this.
5. This automatic action keeps the eyeball moist.

8.1.10. Clue Word: President

TOPIC SENTENCE: Andrew Johnson, instead of being sent to school, was apprenticed to a tailor and continued to make his own suits even when serving as the seventeenth President of the United States.

CLUE SENTENCES:

1. Who was Andrew Johnson?
2. What is an apprentice?
3. To what trade was he apprenticed?
4. Did he follow his trade when he became President of the United States?

8.1.11. Clue Word: Kite

TOPIC SENTENCE: On June 5, 1752, Benjamin Franklin made his famous experiment of sending a kite in the air during a thunderstorm to prove his theory that lightning was electricity.

CLUE SENTENCES:

1. You see lightning during a thunderstorm.
2. Who made a lightning experiment famous?
3. What theory did Benjamin Franklin want to prove?

8.1.12. Clue Words: Eye Teeth*

TOPIC SENTENCE: The canine or eye teeth received their name because their roots are the longest of all our teeth and people believed these teeth extended to the eyes, so if they were removed the person would become blind.

CLUE SENTENCES:

1. What is another name for eye teeth?
2. The roots of our teeth are not all the same length.
3. People often have strange beliefs or superstitions.
4. Do you believe your teeth affect your vision?

---

*Contributed by Roberta Fields and adapted.

*8.1.13. Clue Word: Apples**

TOPIC SENTENCE: Scientists tell us an apple a day might keep the doctor away, for apples do prevent colds and it is possible they even tranquilize you.

CLUE SENTENCES:

1. What do scientists tell us about apples?
2. Do you ever catch cold?
3. Some people use tranquilizers for nervousness.

ADD (in full voice): The old saying "an apple a day keeps the doctor away" is from an old English saying, "Ate an apple avore gwain to bed makes the doctor beg his bread."

8.1.14. Clue Words: Mount Rushmore

TOPIC SENTENCE: The familiar picture of the figures carved from living granite on Mount Rushmore (show picture) in the Black Hills of South Dakota was made with the prediction by Gutzon Borglum that in 100,000 years one inch of stone would erode.

CLUE SENTENCES:

1. Have you ever seen this monument?
2. Where is it?
3. What is the name of the sculptor?
4. What prediction did the sculptor make about the rate of erosion?
5. Can you name the figures on the monument?

8.1.15. Clue Words: Chess

TOPIC SENTENCE: Chess, one of the oldest games in the world, is believed to have been originated more than 5000 years ago in China, Persia, or India.

CLUE SENTENCES:

1. Do you play chess?
2. It is one of the oldest games.
3. How long ago may it have originated?
4. From what countries may it have come?

---

*August 1963 *MD Magazine* and adapted.

ADD (with full voice): A game resembling chess was played over 5000 years ago. It probably originated in China, Persia, or India. The game reached Europe through Persia and Arabia. It was brought to Spain by the Arabs in the eighth century. The word "chess" comes from an old Persian word. The Persian word means "king confounded."

8.1.16. Clue Words: "Mothering Sunday"—simnel

TOPIC SENTENCE: "Mothering Sunday" was celebrated centuries ago in England on the fourth Sunday in Lent with a gift of flowers and a cake made with simnel flour for mother.

CLUE SENTENCES:

1. A century is 100 years.
2. "Mothering Sunday" is an English celebration.
3. How many Sundays are there in Lent?
4. Do you use cake flour when you bake a cake?
5. What is simnel flour?

Back to original topic sentence.

ADD (with more voice if necessary): Simnel is a very fine wheat flour. It is still used today in England for the special "Mothering Sunday" cake. The simnel cake is usually a rich fruit cake frosted with almond paste — sounds delicious!

8.1.17. Clue Word: Leap Year

TOPIC SENTENCE: Every fourth year is leap year, when an extra day is added to the calendar to make the solar year and the calendar year come once more together.

CLUE SENTENCES:

1. Leap year comes every four years.
2. That year an extra day is added to the calendar.
3. 365 days represents a calendar year.
4. $365\frac{1}{4}$ days represents a solar year.

Repeat the original sentence.

EXPLANATION FOR ADDED INTEREST: Can you imagine the confusion we would have if our calendars had $365\frac{1}{4}$ days? Men adjusted the calendar we know to the solar calendar by simply adding one day for every four years. The earth in its orbit does not quite return to the exact same spot after 365 rotations. It would take another one-fourth day to complete the "natural" year. The leap year solves the problem every four years and the two calendars are again in step.

*8.1.18. Clue Word: Margarine**

TOPIC SENTENCE: If you think margarine is a modern product you are wrong, for more than one hundred years ago Napoleon III of France offered a prize for an inexpensive substitute for butter, which turned out to be margarine.

CLUE SENTENCES:

1. Do you ever use margarine?
2. Margarine is not a modern product.
3. Napoleon III was emperor of France over one hundred years ago.
4. Did you ever win a prize?
5. What butter substitute do you use?

Back to original topic sentence.

ADD SHORT STORY FOR ADVANCED STUDENTS: A Frenchman won the prize in 1869. The invention was called margarine, after the Greek word for "pearl-like." The product had a pearly luster when crystallizing. This primitive margarine was not like today's product, but the name persists.

---

*Adapted from *The Herald Examiner,* March 1969.

Chapter 9

PARAGRAPHS FOR COMPREHENSION

Intermediate and Advanced Materials

PARAGRAPHS FOR COMPREHENSION are for intermediate and advanced speechreading instruction. They are an extension of Topic Sentences. The paragraphs are brief information stories. They are a greater challenge to the speechreader for the language is less visible, the words may be unfamiliar, and the vocabulary adult. The student tries to reach a perceptual closure as the subject develops. While these paragraphs are more involved than topic sentences, they are also preliminary to the Stories of Connected Speech, which require longer periods of concentration. The student enjoys greater skill in speechreading. He usually finds these paragraphs offer some new and interesting information while expanding his vocabulary.

PROCEDURE

1. A clue to the general topic is introduced first. This may be done by writing the title on the board. Some stories that include proper names may require additional clues. Proper names should also be written. No further expansion is given.
2. The entire story or paragraph is told without interruption.
3. The reading of the paragraph is followed by questions to clarify the content.
4. After students respond and all have understood, the paragraph is read once more with a more reduced voice.
5. A few sentences in the paragraph are reviewed while the student is auding. These paragraphs lend themselves well to the attentive listening technique.

9.1. FISH COUGH*

This may be of special interest to fishermen. Did you know fish cough? This is a fact discovered by the Environmental Protection Agency. By using polygraphs, fish were monitored. It showed trout normally coughed as often as three times a minute. Sunfish cough about once every five minutes. Why do they cough? The water is contaminated by residues of mercury and copper. When these pollutants get into fresh water they make fish cough. Trout, sunfish, salmon, and blue gills try to rid their gills of debris by coughing. It is just as natural as anyone clearing his throat. If the coughing continues it could be a warning our lakes and streams are becoming more contaminated with pollutants.

QUESTIONS:

1. What does EPA stand for?
2. What has the agency discovered?
3. What makes fish cough?
4. Is it unusual for fish to cough?
5. What can we learn from this study?

9.2. CONTACT LENS*

Would you be surprised to know the contact lens is not a modern invention? The principle of the first contact lens was theorized by Leonardo da Vinci in the fifteenth century. Since then many others have suggested ways to improve vision by placing a device on the cornea. About the middle of the twentieth century contact lens were greatly improved. They were made of light weight plastic. They have continued to improve since then and now a soft lens is available. It is approved by the Food and Drug Administration. The soft lens looks like a button (blob) of clear Jello®. It is made of a plastic that absorbs water, which makes it easy to wear. Most people are able to wear the soft lens from the first moment it is placed in the eye.

QUESTIONS:

1. Are contact lenses a completely new invention?

---

*Adapted from an article in the *Los Angeles Times,* 1974.

*Adapted from an article in *Family Health,* 1972.

2. Who was responsible for the idea of the contact lens?
3. When did Leonardo da Vinci live?
4. What improvement has been made for the contact lens.
5. Can you describe what a soft lens looks like?

9.3. WHY IS IT CALLED RUBBER"?*

Note: The teacher should place the proper names on the board. Say them with and without voice with student response.

Hernando Cortez	conquistador
Joseph Priestley	chemist

Hernando Cortez was the Spanish conqueror of Mexico. When he came to the New World, he discovered something unknown to Spain. It was a peculiar property of a tree. This tree produced a gum. When formed into a ball, it bounced. A practical use for this new material was discovered by Joseph Priestly, an English chemist. He used a piece of the gum to rub out some pencil marks. It worked much better than bread crumbs, the usual substance for erasing marks. Mr. Priestly called it "rubber."

QUESTIONS:

1. Who discovered the gumlike substance?
2. What was peculiar about a ball of the stuff?
3. Who was Joseph Priestley?
4. Why did he call it rubber?

9.4. WORM FIDDLING, CARYVILLE, FLORIDA†

Every July there is a special celebration held in Florida. The small community of Caryville hosts the International Worm Fiddling Contest. There is a definite procedure for fiddling up a worm. A stake is driven into the ground. Then another stake is rubbed across the top. The ground vibrates and the worms come to the surface. Spectators and bettors are there for the contest. Trophies are awarded. One trophy is given for the greatest number of worms fiddled up. Another trophy is presented for the

---

*Adapted from an article in *MD Magazine,* November 1972.

†Adapted from an article in *The Old Farmer's Almanac,* 1974.

largest single worm. Why have a contest like this? It's for the purpose of getting worms for fishing, of course.

QUESTIONS:

1. When does this event take place?
2. What is the full name of the event?
3. Describe worm fiddling.
4. What awards are given?

9.5. STREAKING*

When streaking began in 1973 everyone was surprised. It began at the University of Florida and the University of Maryland. It spread fast. Before long thousands of students all over the United States were streaking. But not all streakers were students. A banker streaked down Wall Street. In Paris, tourists streaked under the Eiffel Tower. At West Point, cadets streaked across the parade ground. They were followed by furious officers in uniform. Streakers were everywhere. Someone streaked through a 747 jet going to London. In Alaska, some streakers ran through eight-degree weather. They wore boots and snow caps. Why do people streak? One man said, "To keep the world safe for goldfish." (That remark borrowed from grandfather's day may have to be explained to the young people.) Streaking will be remembered as one of the shortest-lived fads of our times.

QUESTIONS:

1. When and where did streaking begin?
2. Name some place where a person streaked.
3. How cold was it in Alaska?
4. How will streaking be remembered?

9.6. A TAIL IMPLANT*

Today transplants are quite commonplace in the world of medicine. Now, thanks to skilled doctors of the University of Minnesota, a wounded falcon was given a tail implant. It was perhaps the first peregrine falcon to have the "operation." A

---

*Contributed by Maresa Molinar.

*Adapted from an article in the *Minneapolis Tribune*, Minneapolis, Minnesota.

female falcon had been shot and her wing was broken. She rubbed off the tail feathers while recuperating in a veterinarian's cage. The transplanting process is called "imping." Small pieces of bamboo were put inside some donated feathers. Then doctors attached the feathers to the stubs in the tail. They were secured with quick-drying glue. Eventually the falcon would have grown feathers to replace the lost ones. The operation was done because the bird had forgotten how to fly. To wait so long for new feathers would mean keeping her too long in captivity. She then would probably not be able to cope with life in the wild again. A falcon expert gave her some flight training. Now she flies in freedom along the Rio Grande in Texas.

QUESTIONS:

1. What bird received the implant?
2. What was the process called?
3. Describe the "operation."
4. Why was it necessary?

Chapter 10

STORIES OF CONNECTED SPEECH

Information, Narration, Description, and Humorous Stories

THE STORIES OF CONNECTED SPEECH are perhaps the most difficult exercise in the progression from beginning to advanced speechreading skill. At the same time the story is the most satisfying as a conclusion to a lesson. The speechreader can be more relaxed to follow the continuing sequence of thought without the pressure of being called upon for answers. An interesting informative story provides a child with something to share at home or at school, a psychological boost. The adult also benefits, for he frequently contributes additional information on the subject. It has been this teacher's experience to have her program enriched with the shared knowledge of her students.

The Stories of Connected Speech have important values for the speechreader.

1. It takes the pressure off. He is less dependent on instant knowledge as to the correctness of his speechreading.
2. It forces the reader to depend on contextual clues, not to give up if he misses a fragment. He must "hang in there" until the gap closes and his mind has filled in what he believed he missed. This does occur for the speechreader, to his eternal gratitude.
3. Vision and auding usually results in improvement in two important skills. First, the ability to retain visual imagery, which he could not immediately identify. Secondly, the ability to recall what was read to him. There should always be a time following the reading of a long story for a pupil to ask for

anything he believed he missed or cannot remember.

The teacher has an added responsibility when giving this kind of story. Great care and preparation goes into the lesson to keep the language as visible as possible and the ideas or associational clues flowing for a satisfactory story experience. The story of connected speech is a great help to wean the "must-see-every-word" pupil. He learns not every word in a conversation will *always* be seen. We should say *ever* be seen. He should get the essence and enjoy.

These stories are referred to as enrichment material. The subject matter is probably not found in most school curricula. Included are stories of description, narration, humor, as well as information.

There are several ways of introducing the lessons. One is to discuss the subject from which the story is adapted. A skillful teacher may direct and structure the discussion in preparation for the story. In many of the lessons in this book the discussion precedes an orientation, which clearly sets the story content. There is a difference to be noted between the discussion of the topic where both teacher and students contribute something pertinent to the subject, and the orientation or introduction. The latter is a brief preface to the story which is *always given with full voice.*

After an orientation a teacher may use a second approach, that of introducing clue words. The words are written on the board in the sequential order in which they appear in the story. They give a mental set to the story content, making it possible for the pupil to better anticipate the development of the information. Clue words should be gone over first with voice then at random selection without voice. Clue sentences which further extend the information preliminary to the main body of the story may follow the clue words. Not all stories need both approaches.

Whenever possible visual aids should be used in the form of pictures, maps, or objects. A story may well be given with only visual aids. It would depend on the complexity of the vocabulary and the ability of the speechreader. Stories should be given with some voice. In the presentation there could be no voice for very brief periods of time. This precludes a tendency to listen without looking momentarily. An effective device is to emphasize with more sound a word in a sentence that is obscure visually. The added vowel energy could provide a perceptual link in an otherwise lost sentence. The instructor must be familiar with the story, never looking down at a script. He must be telling, not reading, the story. A brief retelling of a portion of any story gives emphasis to the Look and Listen method. The student is exposed to a longer period of recall and information through auditory channels.

The first stories in this section are suitable for young children. The later stories are for older children, teenagers, and adults. The teacher will find many of these stories are easily reduced and adapted for young children.

10.1. STORIES FOR CHILDREN

10.1.1. Activity Story—Building a House

PROCEDURE: Draw a large rectangle on the board to represent the house. Instruct elementary students where to put the objects after asking each question and receiving an answer.

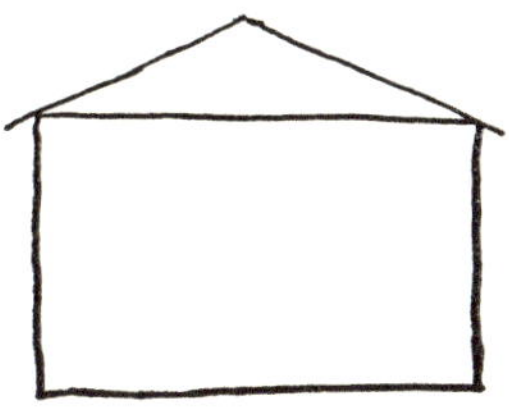

What keeps the rain out of the house?
Put the roof on the house.

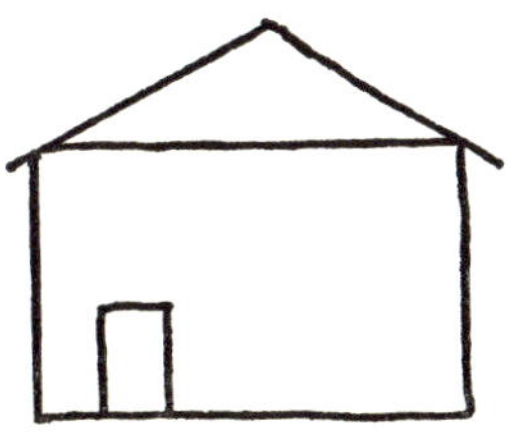

How do you get into the house?
Place the door on the left front side.

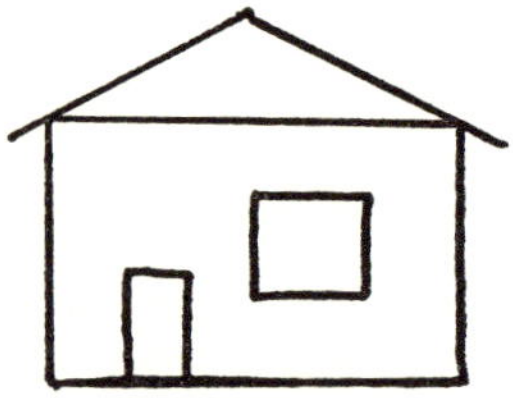

What lets the light in?
Put a window in front of the house.

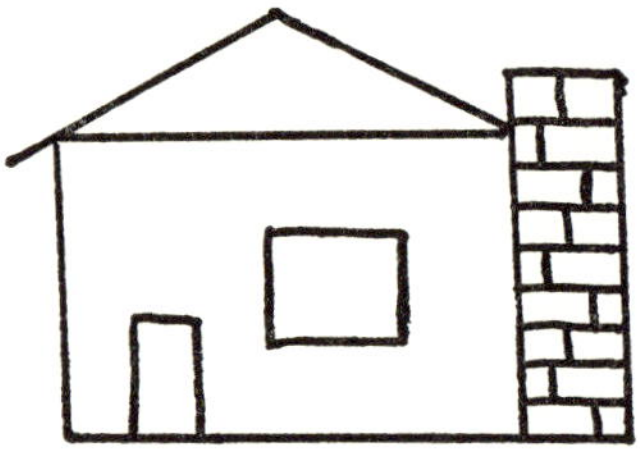

How does the smoke get out of the house?
Put the chimney on the right-hand side of the house.

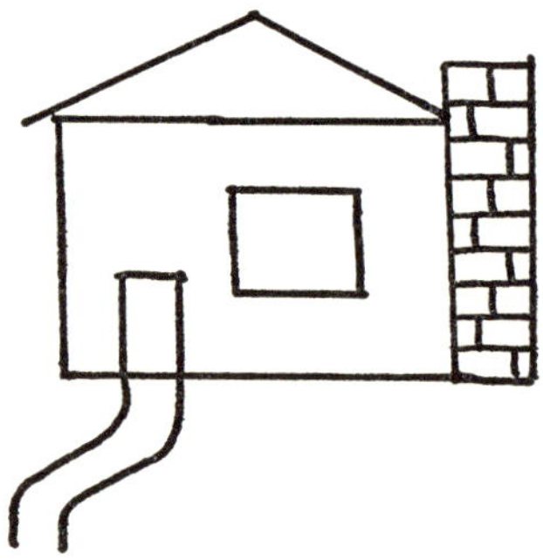

How do you get up to the house?
Put the sidewalk up to the front door.

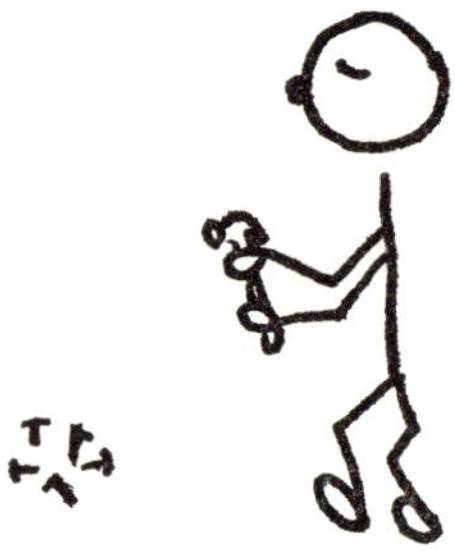

Who builds the house?
Put nails beside the carpenter.
Put a hammer in his hand.

Follow the story with the *Quiz: House* in Section 11.1.2.

10.1.2.—A Mystery Story—About the Five Senses

Visual Aids: One large chart picturing each of the senses: see, hear, smell, taste, and touch. Five smaller separate charts each picturing one sense. A box containing a bell.

Procedure: The story is given in reduced voice. The chart with the five senses is shown when the principals in the story are introduced as a group. The same procedure is followed when each sense and the box is mentioned separately. The box is shaken when Mr. Ear "hears" it.

*Story**

This is a mystery story.
There are five detectives in the story.
They will try to solve the mystery.
The names of the detectives are Mr. Eye, Mr. Ear, Mr. Nose, Mr. Skin, and Mr. Tongue.
This is a mysterious box.
What is inside this box?

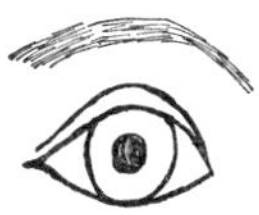

Mr. Eye looks, but cannot see in it.

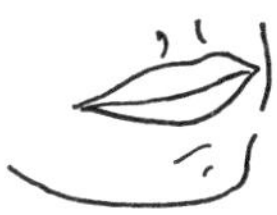

Mr. Tongue tries, but cannot taste it.

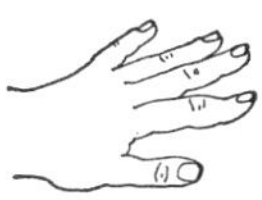

Mr. Skin touches, but cannot feel what is in the box.

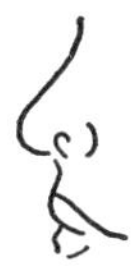

Mr. Nose sniffs but cannot smell anything.

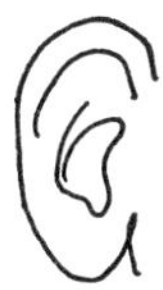

But Mr. Ear shakes the box. He can hear something.

*Contributed by Melba V. Brown and adapted.

Mr. Ear says, "It's a ______!" (allow for spontaneous answer).

Let the student who answers first shake the box and tell the story to the class. The story may be followed by the *Quiz: Five Senses* in Section 11.1.3.

10.1.3. Information Story—Animal Families

The lesson names the animal, father, mother, baby, and group. Most of the terms are familiar with occasional unfamiliar terms introduced.

VISUAL AIDES: Pictures of the animals.

PROCEDURE: Show the picture or pictures of one group. Get student responses identifying and naming members of the animal group. Write the names on the board under each classification. Give the information and ask a student to tell in his own words what was said.

Clue Words: Write on the board the classification: *Animal—Father—Mother—Baby—Group* (Family)

Story

The bee is called an animal or an insect. The father of a bee is a drone. Every bee has a queen for a mother! The baby has no other name except "bee." The family lives in a hive. When bees are flying in a group we say they are in a swarm.

Chickens are called fowls as well as animals. The father is a rooster. The mother is a hen. A chick is a baby. Chicks are soft and yellow with big eyes. Many chickens together are a flock.

Deer are beautiful wild animals. The baby is called a fawn. A mother deer is a doe. The father is called a buck or stag. He wears antlers or horns. The fawns have spotted coats. This is a camouflage and protects them from other wild animals. A herd is a large group of deer.

Some say the fox is a sly animal. The father is called Reynard. That is a French word for fox. Vixen is the name for a mother. Babies have three names: pup, cub, and kit. The name for a group of foxes is a skulk.

The goose has been called "silly." But all geese are very intelligent (smart). The father is called a gander. A baby goose is a gosling. The female is just mother goose! Geese live together in flocks or gaggles. When geese are flying in a group it is a skein.

The goat family is valuable to us. It gives us wool and milk. The name for a father is a buck. A mother goat is a doe. Kids are baby goats. They are playful and make good pets. Many goats are a herd or a trip.

Everyone knows the horse. Horses work for us and give us pleasure. A baby horse is a foal, not a pony. The mother horse is a mare. The father is called a stallion. They live in stables unless they are wild; then they are called herds of horses.

The kangaroo family was first found in Australia. Mother kangaroo is called a doe or flyer. She carries her baby in a pouch. The baby is called a joey. Father kangaroo is a buck or a boomer. The group name is troop or herd.

There are more lions in Africa than in any other country. The father is called a lion and the mother is a lioness. Baby lions are cubs. They are as playful as kittens. Lions hunt their food in clans, but a family living together is called a pride.

Do you have a rabbit for a pet? Baby rabbits are called kittens. Buck is the name for the father. Mother rabbit is a doe. The group of rabbits is a colony. Sometimes a group is called a warren.

Follow with the *Game of Recall,* Section 11.1.4.

*10.1.4. Wilbur Woodpecker's Adventure**

PROCEDURE: Write the title on the board.

The teacher asks: "Do you know what an adventure is?"

Allow for some discussion.

The teacher may then introduce words or ideas which will help establish the forthcoming vocabulary, such as fun, exciting, and living in a tree.

VISUAL AIDS: Pictures of woodpeckers and trees indicating holes where birds enter nests.

CLUE SENTENCES:

1. Have you ever seen a woodpecker?
2. How do you think it got its name?

---

*Contributed by Vannah Vannoy and adapted.

3. Wilbur wanted to have an adventure.
4. Listen to Wilbur's adventure.

Story

Wilbur Woodpecker lived in an old tree with his father and mother.

His home was in a hole in an old tree.

Wilbur liked to look out of the hole and watch birds flying to other trees.

He wanted to join them and have an adventure.

Flying looked like fun.

But his mother and father said he must stay in the family tree.

Some day he would be old enough to fly away.

One day Wilbur decided he was old enough.

So he hopped out of the nest and flew to another tree.

He chirped and chirped bird talk with the other birds.

It was the most fun he had ever had.

Wilbur started for home and stopped to rest on the roof of a house.

He pecked and pecked on the wood.

This was really exciting and made a lot of noise.

Now Wilbur did not know anything about people.

He saw a man run out of the house.

He had a long, shiny stick.

It made a terrible noise. BANG!

Wilbur was frightened and flew home fast.

His mother said, "What happened to your beautiful tail feather?"

Wilbur said, "A big bang blew it off. I am glad to be back in our family tree. Adventures are scary."

QUESTIONS:

1. Why did Wilbur want to leave the family tree?
2. What was fun for Wilbur?
3. Where did he stop to rest on the way home?
4. Why do you think the man was angry?
5. What was the long, shiny stick that Wilbur saw?
6. What happened?
7. What did he tell his parents?

Retell portions of the story with full voice while the students listen only.

10.1.5. Santa Claus' Picture

VISUAL AIDS: Pictures of Santa Claus, including a copy of the original drawing by Thomas Nast.

Clue Words (placed on the board preceding the story):

cartoonist	laughing	beard	solemn
Thomas Nast	toys	jolly	image
Bavaria	switches	popular	

Story

Who gave us a picture of Santa Claus?
It was a famous cartoonist.
His name was Thomas Nast.
He was born in Bavaria in 1840.
The children in Bavaria believed in an old fellow who came at Christmas with gifts.
He gave toys to good children.
He brought switches to bad ones.
He was thin and not a laughing old man.
Thomas Nast came to America when he was six years old.
He remembered the old man of his childhood days.
When he was a man he drew pictures for books.
He wanted children in America to have a happy Christmas.
He drew the old fellow with a beard and changed the way he looked.
He made him fat, jolly, and laughing instead of solemn.
His Santa Claus pictures became popular right away.
His picture is known in most of the world.
The image we all have of Santa Claus was made more than one hundred years ago.
Santa Claus will never grow older to children everywhere.

*10.1.6. Hot Doughnuts**

My mother used to bake delicious doughnuts. She always put them in a big cookie jar in the kitchen. Mother found it difficult

*Contributed by Virignia M. Moore and adapted.

to keep the jar filled. Everyone liked her doughnuts so much. Especially my cousin. My cousin never asked for doughnuts. He just took as many as he wanted without asking. Sometimes he would come over when no one was home. He would help himself to the doughnuts and leave the jar empty. This made my mother mad so she decided to teach him a lesson. One day she made a very special doughnut. This doughnut was full of hot chili powder. But, it looked the same as all the others. She put it on top of the pile of fresh doughnuts. When my cousin came over that day, he went right to the cookie jar. As usual, he took one without asking. He picked the top doughnut. The one that was full of chili powder! What a surprise he had when he bit into it! Can you imagine how it tasted? Do you think he ever ate my mother's doughnuts again? Not without asking! He'd learned his lesson, thanks to that hot chili powder!

10.2. STORIES FOR OLDER CHILDREN AND ADULTS

10.2.1. The Crow

PROCEDURE: The story is introduced with clue words and clue sentences for an intermediate group. An advanced class may need only one or the other.

VISUAL AIDS: Pictures of the crow and scarecrows.

Orientation (full voice): The crow is perhaps the best-known bird in our country. It is found north of Florida to the Arctic and west to the arid plains. No one especially wants the crow on his property, and it is not protected wherever it lives. But if anyone should call you a "birdbrain," hope he means the crow, for the crow is extremely intelligent.

Clue Words on Board

glossy	thief	clannish
raucous	grain	sentimental
laws	mischief	insects
habits	tame	Aesop

CLUE SENTENCES:

1. Another word for glossy is shiny.
2. Raucous means noisy and harsh.

3. Laws are made for protection.
4. There are good and bad habits.
5. The crow has been called a thief.
6. The clan is a social group.
7. A sentinel watches over a group.
8. Can you name an insect that is a pest?
9. What kind of stories did Aesop tell?

Story

The crow is a large black bird. He is about twenty inches long. He belongs to the same family as the Blue Jay. He has glossy plummage. His voice has been called raucous. Everyone seems to be against the crow. There are no laws to protect it. This is because the crow has some habits we do not like. The farmer will tell you he is a thief. He steals small birds, eggs, and young chickens. He pulls up sprouting corn and other grains. The farmer makes scarecrows to keep them out of corn fields. The crow is forever stirring up mischief. He will run off with small, shiny objects and hide them. Some are easy to tame and can be trained to talk.

Crows are clannish. They live in large groups and have a sentinel to guard them. The sentinel gives signals to warn of danger. Crows seem to have a large vocabulary and often meet for bird-talk. They are not all bad! Crows destroy large amounts of insect pests. They are devoted parents. They take very good care of their babies, who seem to be hungry all the time. The babies eat so much it takes both mother and father to keep them fed. They build safe homes high in trees. Crows have been called very intelligent. Aesop told a fable many hundreds of years ago about how a clever crow got a drink of water. Do you know this story? (The Crow and the Pitcher)

Questions:

1. Can you describe the crow?
2. Why is the crow disliked?
3. How do crows live?
4. What are some good points about the crow?
5. Where do they nest?

6. How long has the crow been known?

CROW EXPRESSIONS: Here are some expressions we have borrowed from our knowledge of the crow.

1. to crow over	means to boast and be loud while bragging.
2. as the crow flies	means the shortest and most direct route.
3. to eat crow	means to apologize and admit a mistake.
4. a scarecrow	means someone bad enough looking to be frightening.
5. an old crow	means someone loud and noisy.
6. crows-feet	means unwanted wrinkles around the eyes that look like shape of the feet of a crow.
7. crow's nest	is a name for a lookout point or a high perch.

*10.2.2. The Tornado Warning**

My friend moved from California to Oklahoma City. One of her biggest surprises was that Oklahoma had tornados. Her only tornado experience came from watching the *Wizard of Oz*. Because this was all so new, she wanted to know what to prepare in case of a tornado. The place where she lived didn't have a cellar. The next best thing was to open the window farthest from the tornado. Then, one should get his mattress and pull it into the bathroom. Finally, jump into the bathtub and pull the mattress over yourself. One night, not long after learning the preparations, my friend and her husband were watching television. The program was interrupted and a "tornado watch" was announced. Frightened, they grabbed their mattress and jumped into the tub. They waited for a long time. Finally the phone rang. My friend bravely climbed from the tub to answer it. It was one of her friends. He couldn't stop laughing when he learned what they had done. Tornado watches in Oklahoma City were as common as rain.

*Contributed by Jan Ganong and adapted.

10.2.3. How Many Donkeys Are There?

This story for intermediate speechreaders is introduced with only clue words.

Clue Words

Abool		wheat	sacks
India	mill	counted	climbed

*Story**

Abool was a farmer in India. He lived in a small village with seven other farmers. They raised wheat. They could not grind the wheat themselves. They had to take the wheat to the mill to be ground into flour. The farmers used donkeys to carry the wheat to the mill. One day it was Abool's turn to take the wheat to the mill. Abool put the sacks of wheat on the donkeys. Then he counted the donkeys. There were one, two, three, four, five, six, seven, eight donkeys. Abool climbed on the first donkey and started for the mill. After a while he counted the donkeys. There were only seven. "Someone has stolen a donkey," said Abool. He got off his donkey and looked for the missing donkey. When he came back, there were eight donkeys! "I don't understand this. I counted the donkeys myself," he said. Abool got back on his donkey and counted them again, one, two, three four, five, six, seven. There were only seven donkeys. Abool again looked for the missing donkey. When he came back there were eight donkeys. Abool was confused. When Abool got to the mill he told the miller that someone kept taking a donkey and bringing it back. The miller laughed and laughed. He told Abool there were really nine donkeys. He told Abool to look in a mirror and he could see the ninth donkey. Abool saw himself in the mirror. The miller said that Abool had forgotten to count the donkey he was sitting on.

*10.2.4. Eyes**

The story develops through single-word clues, simple draw-

*Contributed by Barbara Steadman, adapted from an old fable for children.

*Adapted from *Walters Comparative Anatomy*. Expanded information provided by Earl L. Lewis, M.D., San Marino, California.

ings, statements, and questions by the teacher. The students answer from prepared slips, making this a participation lesson. The format differs from the others described in the text. It is suited for better speechreaders.

VISUAL AIDS: Pictures of each of the animal life in the story or simple drawings placed on the board as each one is discussed.

PROCEDURE:

1. Orientation, full voice.
2. A single clue word is given with greatly reduced voice. A volunteer gives the word to the class with voice. The word is written on the board.
3. An illustration is shown or a picture drawn of the organism or animal.
4. The teacher gives briefly some information describing it (reduced voice). A response from a student or students, with voice, repeats the teacher's statements.
5. A question (about the eyes of the named animal) is asked by the teacher. A student with the written information gives it, with reduced voice, in front of the class.

Orientation (full voice): The hard-of-hearing and deaf persons are especially aware of their dependency on eyes. The eyes must augment the ears. So perhaps these people are even more interested than others in the history of the beginning of eyes. The development of sight from one-celled organisms to the complex and wonderful eyesight given to humans is a fascinating story. This is a short story of how eyes began.

Story

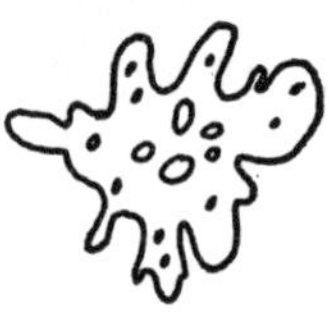

The word amobea comes from the German word meaning "change." This is what the amoeba does. It is in a constant change of shape. The amoeba is called the lowest form of animal life.

Question: Does the amoeba have an organ for seeing?

Answer: The amoeba has no special organ for seeing. But it can tell the difference between light and dark.

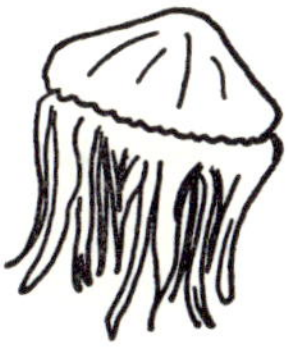

In spite of its name, the jellyfish is not like a fish. It does not have fins or a long body covered with scales. It has a few feelers or tentacles which hang down below its umbrella-shaped body. It is one of the most unusual of sea animals.

Question: Does it have eyes?

Answer: The jellyfish was the first to have eyes. The eyes are around the edge of the umbrella top of the jellyfish. They are called simple eyes. They cannot see shape or form.

The starfish is another sea animal that is not a fish. It is a sea animal with five arms which make it look like a star. The starfish is found in waters all over the world except the polar regions.

Question: What are the "eyes" of the starfish?

Answer: The "eyes" of the starfish are simply a group of cells that are sensitive to light.

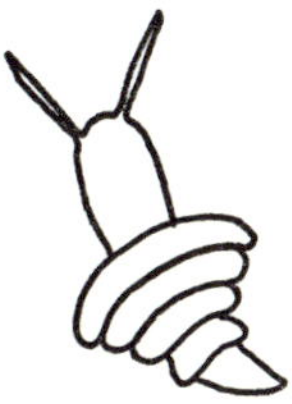

The snail is a mollusk. It is a sea animal living in a shell. The snail was the first to have a cornea. The cornea is the clear, transparent part that covers the eye. The cornea lets light through to the eye.

Question: Where is the eye of a snail?

Answer: The eye of the snail is on the end of the long horn or tentacle that comes out of its head. The snail has a great advantage over most animals. If it should lose one of its "eye horns" another will grow in its place.

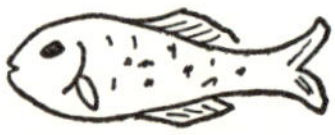

Fish were the first to have an eye equipped with a lens. The lens of fish is movable. A fish has to move its eyes back and forth to focus sharply. A fish does not have eyelids because it doesn't need them to keep its eyes moist and clean. But fish have an eye problem.

Question: What problem do fish have that is the same as a human might have?

Answer: Fish are nearsighted. Fish can see only objects close to them. Authorities say fish can see different colors. Ask any fisherman. He will tell you fish are attracted to color.

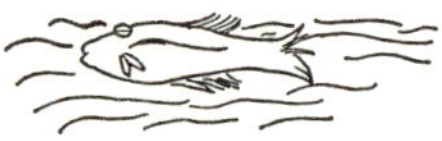

There are strange fish living in rivers in South and Central America. They swim on the surface of the water.

Question: What is unusual about their eyes?

Answer: Their eyes are divided across the center. There is a black line that runs horizontally across the eyes. They can see both above and below water at the same time.

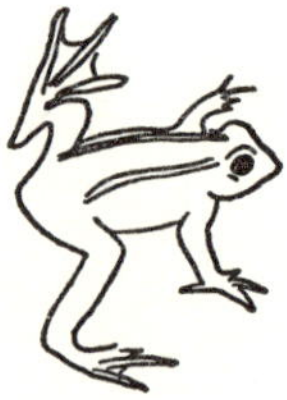

Amphibians are animals that live a double life. They are able to live both on land and in water. Frogs and toads are amphibians.

Question: When the animals moved out of the water, they had a problem. What was it?

Answer: Their problem was they were getting dust in the eyes. They had no way of removing dust particles. So nature gave them tear ducts (more voice) to keep the eyes clean. Amphibians were the first animals to be given tear ducts.

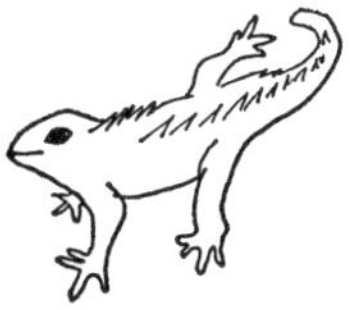

The sphenodon (sfí-no-don) is a reptile. This reptile is a lizard-like creature. It is found in New Zealand. It looks much like the iguana.

Question: What is unusual about its eyes?

Answer: The sphenodon has three eyes. The third eye is in the back of its head. The reptile does not see with this eye. It is simply a kind of socket or "eye-like" formation.

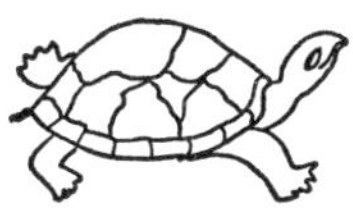

The turtle had the first iris. There are muscles in the iris of the eye. These muscles regulate the amount of light that enters the eye. The iris can become narrow to keep out light, or widen to allow more light to enter.

Question: What can happen to give a turtle poor eyesight?

Answer: A turtle must have sunlight and good food for good eyesight. Without them the turtle's eyes will swell shut.

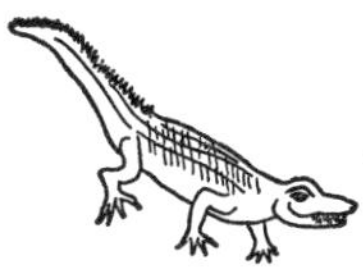

An alligator is called the American crocodile. The name for an alligator is vertebrate. It was the first vertebrate to have a flexible lens.

Question: How does a flexible lens help the alligator to see?

Answer: The flexible lens helps the alligator to focus the eyes more sharply on an object. Their eyes adjust easily to things nearby or in the distance.

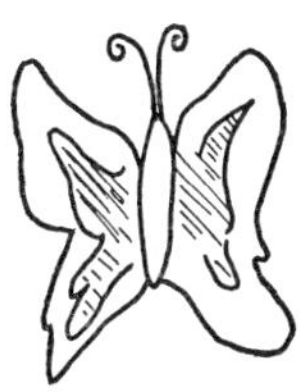

Many insects have more than one pair of eyes. Some of these insects are butterflies, moths, bees, and ants.

Question: How are the eyes of butterflies and moths described?

Answer: The eyes of butterflies and moths are described as compound. This means they are made up of many individual seeing parts. These eyes are large and well developed.

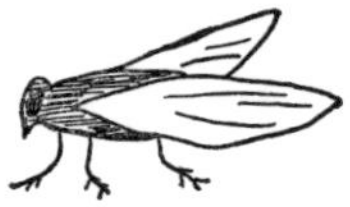

A fly is an insect that is hard to catch. It always seems to see you coming with a swatter.

Question: Does a fly have sharp vision?

Answer: A fly has five eyes. Two of these are so large they cover most of its head. These are compound eyes. Between them are three tiny simple eyes. But with all the eyes, a fly does not have sharp vision.

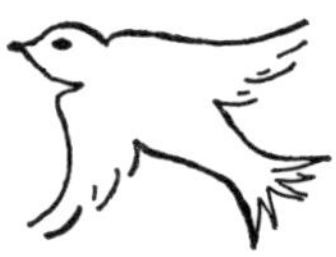

All birds have extremely sharp vision. They are farsighted. The eyesight of birds is more sharp than a human's vision. They are said to have the most efficient eyes in the animal kingdom.

Question: What kind of vision do owls and hawks have?

Answer: Owls and hawks have binocular vision. They look straightforward with both eyes together. But they are able to look off to the sides using each eye independent of the other.

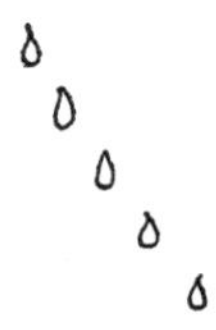

Birds have color vision. It has been found that birds see color. Nature has provided birds with very tiny drops of oil in their eyes. It is belived that these tiny oil drops are responsible for color vision of birds.

Question: What colors are in the oil?

Answer: The oil in birds' eyes seems to be red, orange, yellow, and at times, blue and green. Higher animals do not have these drops of oil in their eyes.

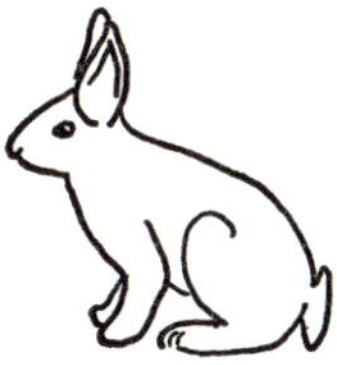

Some animals are not able to fight their enemies very well. So nature has given them the ability to see the slightest motion to help them escape. A rabbit is one of these animals. Its eyes are very sensitive to motion.

Question: Describe the eyes of a rabbit.

Answer: Rabbits have large eyes. Each eye is able to see more than a half-circle. With both eyes a rabbit can see in every direction. A rabbit can watch for a hawk in the air. At the same time, he can spot a rock or a bush to hide under.

Conclude (with voice): Nature has provided all its creatures with eyes suited to their environment. We have only one pair of eyes. Take care of them.

*10.2.5. Distance in Outer Space**

Part I

Clue Words

distance	trillion
outer space	billion
light years	

CLUE SENTENCES:

1. The distance between two objects is the amount of space between them.
2. Someday we may travel in outer space.
3. Light years is an easy way to measure distance in outer space.
4. Trillion is a number we don't hear very often.
5. Billion is a smaller number than trillion.

Story

How far is it from New York to San Francisco? (3032 miles). It is easy for us to think about distance in terms of miles, but what about distance in outer space? We measure distance in

*Contributed by Russell Harvey.

outer space in units of light years. A light year is the distance that light travels in one year or $365\frac{1}{4}$ days. Light travels at the rate of about 186,000 miles per second. This is about 5 trillion, 880 billion miles a year. So this figure represents a light year.

QUESTIONS:

1. How do we measure distance in outer space?
2. How fast does light travel in one second?
3. How fast does light travel in one year?

Part II

Clue Words

earth	star
equator	galaxy
sun	Proxima Centauri

CLUE SENTENCES:

1. Earth is the planet on which we live.
2. The equator divides the earth in half.
3. The sun is one of many stars in our galaxy.
4. The sun is our nearest star.
5. Proxima Centauri is the name of one of our stars.

Story

The distance around the earth at the equator is 25,000 miles. If you traveled around the earth in a car at the rate of sixty miles per hour, your trip would take about seventeen days. Now the sun is 93 million (use full voice to avoid confusion with billion) miles from the earth. If you could travel to the sun by car at the rate of sixty miles per hour it would take you 177 years. Suppose you were to take one of our big jet airliners, travelling at six hundred miles per hour, it would still take you seventeen years to reach the sun.

Let's stop and think again how fast light travels. In the time a watch makes a one-second tick, light can travel around the earth more than seven times. Light travelling the 93 million miles from the sun to the earth takes about eight minutes. Our nearest star, other than the sun, is called Proxima Centauri. Light travelling to the earth from this star takes over four years to complete the trip. So we say that the star Proxima Centauri is four light years from the earth. This is about 25 trillion, 222 billion miles.

QUESTIONS:

1. What is the distance around the earth at the equator?
2. How far is the sun from the earth?
3. What is the name of our nearest star, other than the sun?
4. How many trillion miles is four light years?

*10.2.6. The Princess and the Frog**

Introduce this story by a few remarks about the fairy tale of The Princess and The Frog. The format suggested is for students to work in groups of four, simulating a conversational situation. This is a different method of presentation for a story of connected speech. The complete story is written on four slips numbered I to IV. Begin with I and follow in sequential order to the completion of the story. All participants should use a reduced voice. Each group of four students is given the entire story.

I. First Person

One day the fair young Princess was walking through the forest.
As she was walking, she heard a little voice say, "Please stop."
She looked around, but no one was in sight.
She started to take another step.
Then, the little voice said, "Please don't step on me."

II. Second Person

Again, she looked for the voice.
She saw a frog near her feet.
"Are you speaking to me," she asked?
The frog replied, "Yes."
"You see, I am a Prince, or was, until the wicked witch cast a spell on me."

III. Third Person

"Now, I must stay a frog until a Princess will let me spend the night on her pillow."

*Contributed by Roberta Fields and adapted.

"Will you help me?"
"Of course," said the Princess.
She picked the frog up and took him home with her.
That night, when she went to sleep, she put the frog on her pillow.

IV. Fourth Person

In the morning the Queen Mother came to wake the Princess.
When she entered the room, she was surprised at what she saw.
There, not only was the Princess, but beside her the handsome Prince.
Both the Princess and the Prince told the Queen Mother what happened.
Do you know that even today the Queen Mother does not believe their story?

VARIATION: The story may be read by four students sitting in a semicircle in front of the class. Using this arrangement the class will observe each of the four speakers in the semicircle from different angles.

*10.2.7. A Story of Popcorn**

ORIENTATION (with full voice): A baseball game or a movie is not complete without popcorn. It is one of the most primitive fiesta foods known to man. Researchers have found records of popcorn used in pagan religious rites. Archeologists say radiocarbon tests of some found in New Mexico's Bat Cave show it to be 5,600 years old.

Part I

Clue Words

primitive	clay	wholesale
rays	stones	production
sand	electric	crop

Story

Popcorn has been known a long, long time. Primitive man first found it. It was a strange grain that exploded with heat.

*Adapted from an article in the *National Observer,* April 22, 1962.

Possibly the first explosions were the result of the sun's rays. Then corn was probably popped in hot sand in dishes made of clay. Possibly corn popping was done on fireplace stones. And now we have electric poppers at home. There are fully automatic wholesale poppers in mass-popping kitchens. Popcorn production is the second largest crop in our nation's history.

Part II

Clue Words

million	mechanical	kernels
grows	rollers	unpopped
tractor	shelled	per cent

Story

Popcorn production is now over 400 million pounds of ear corn per year. It grows best in the midwest. It is planted with tractor-drawn planters. It is harvested by mechanical pickers. These pickers are equipped with special rollers to grab the smaller ears. Then it is machine-shelled. The kernels are fanned clean. It is polished, fumigated, and packaged for home use or firms that do the popping. The unpopped corn must be absolutely clean. About 50 percent of the crop goes to the home kitchen. A great amount goes to the movies and ball games.

Part III

Clue Words

correct	devil	steam
problems	modern	pressure
ancients	horny starch	cooked

Story

Popcorn must have the correct moisture content for popping. If it is too moist or too dry it won't pop well. This is one of the problems of the processor. The correct moisture content is 11 to 15 percent. What makes popcorn pop? Some ancients believe there was a devil in each kernel. He blew his top when he got hot! Modern scientists explain it this way. Popcorn is a very hard grain. It is composed of what is called horny starch. The heat builds up steam from the moisture in the corn. The moisture is held under terrific pressure before it breaks through the layers of starch. When it does break through, the grain of corn turns inside out. The grain is cooked in the same process.

Part IV

Clue Words

Columbus	statues	detached
Cortez	Spaniard	French explorers
Aztec Indians	Peruvian	Iroquois
	Paraguay	

Story

History has recorded popcorn. Columbus arrived in the West Indies in 1492. He found natives wearing popcorn like corsages. In 1519 Cortez found Aztec Indians wearing popcorn garlands on their ceremonial headdresses. The Aztecs also decorated their statues with popcorn. In 1650 a Spaniard wrote about Peruvian Indians. These Indians used "a corn that burst as a confection." From Paraguay popcorn was described as an interesting corn which was popped without being detached. Early French explorers were in the Great Lakes region in 1612. They found the Iroquois Indians popping corn in pottery with heated sand. At the first Thanksgiving, one account mentioned popped corn. It was brought to the feast by the Indians.

CONCLUDE (with voice): According to the account of the feast, the corn was brought already popped, no doubt done over their familiar campfire. They probably doubted the settlers would know how to pop it!

True, False Statements following Popcorn Story

T 1. Primitive man first found grain that popped.
T 2. Popcorn first popped as a result of sun's rays.
F 3. Next it was popped in fireplaces in clay dishes.
T 4. Electric poppers used today are found in homes and mass kitchens.
F 5. Popcorn production is the largest crop in the nation.

F 6. 400 million pounds of shelled corn are produced annually.
F 7. It grows best in the South.
T 8. It is harvested and shelled by mechanical equipment.
T 9. It is polished, fumigated, and packaged for home use.
F 10. About 40 percent of the crop goes into homes.
F 11. Popcorn will not pop if it is too moist or too dry.
T 12. Indians brought popped corn to the first Thanksgiving feast.

*10.2.8. Famous Women from A to Z**

PROCEDURE: The alphabet is placed on the board in a vertical position, leaving enough room for the students to write a name beside each letter. Slips are made for student participation. Each participant gives the name of the famous person named on his slip, with reduced voice. If the name is not understood, he repeats, using more voice. The name is written beside the letter. The student gives all of the information on his slip. A volunteer repeats what he has understood for the class.

A. Jane Addams

She was an American social worker. She founded Hull House in Chicago. She received the Nobel Peace Prize for her philanthropic work.

B. Evangeline Booth

She is an Englishwoman. She is General of the Salvation Army. She has been Commander of the Army in Canada.

C. Rachel Carson

She was an American scientist. She won several awards for writing. She wrote *Silent Spring,* which was about insecticides.

D. Bette Davis

She is an American actress. She won Academy awards twice for her acting, with 5 nominations. One of the awards was for her work in the film *Jezebel.*

E. Amelia Earhart

She was an American aviatrix. She was the first woman to cross the Atlantic in an airplane. In 1937 she was lost at sea

*Contributed by Dagny Borge.

while on a round-the-world flight.

F. Edna Ferber

She was an American novelist. She began her literary career as a reporter when she was seventeen years old. She was awarded the Pulitzer Prize for her novel *So Big.*

G. Hetty Green

She was an American financier. She inherited a large fortune and managed it shrewdly. She lived like a pauper, but left a fortune estimated to be one hundred million dollars.

H. Sarah Josepha Hale

She was an American editor and author. Mrs. Hale has been called the "Mother of Thanksgiving." She is the one who suggested Thanksgiving be made a national holiday. Her wish was finally granted while Abraham Lincoln was President.

I. Isabella I

She was a Spanish queen. In 1469 she married Ferdinand of Aragon. Queen Isabella financed the explorations of Christopher Columbus.

J. Helen Hunt Jackson

She was a poet and novelist. She published an historical account of the government's injustice to Indians. Her most famous novel was the romance *Ramona.*

K. Helen Keller

She was an American author and lecturer who was blind and deaf. This remarkable woman graduated from Radcliffe College with honors. She spent her lifetime working for the blind.

L. Jenny Lind

She was a well-known and loved Swedish soprano. Under the management of P. T. Barnum she sang in the United States from 1850 to 1852. She was called the "Swedish Nightingale."

M. Maria Montessori

She was an Italian psychiatrist and educator. Her method of education was a modern, "progressive" approach. She believed the child should choose what he wished to learn.

N. Florence Nightingale

She was an English hospital administrator. She organized a hospital unit for the Crimean War. Florence Nightingale is called the "Mother of Nursing."

O. *Georgia O'Keeffe*

She is an American artist. She began her life work illustrating advertisements. She is known for the unusual way she paints flowers.

P. *Anna Pavlova*

She was a Russian ballet dancer. She danced many times in *The Dying Swan*. This ballet was composed for her.

Q. *Queen Marie of Rumania*

She was the granddaughter of Alexander II of Russia and of Queen Victoria of England. She was a Red Cross nurse. She wrote several novels and collections of fairy tales.

R. *Betsy Ross*

She was an American flag-maker. According to legend, she made the first American flag. She is definitely known to have made flags during the American Revolution.

S. *Gertrude Stein*

She was an American author. She studied medicine at Johns Hopkins University. Her style of writing has been called peculiar.

T. *Luisa Tetrazzini*

She was an Italian coloratura soprano. She made her debut in Florence in 1895. Her first American concert was in San Francisco. She appeared with the Metropolitan Opera Company.

U. *Undine*

She is a legendary German water sprite. Her story was written in 1814. The story of Undine is frequently acted in ballet.

V. *Victoria*

She was Queen of England, Great Britain, and Ireland, and Empress of India. She became queen in 1837 when she was eighteen years old. Queen Victoria had the longest reign of any British monarch (64 years).

W. *Ethel Waters*

She was an American singer and actress. She first sang in night clubs and theatres. She wrote *His Eye Is on the Sparrow*, her autobiography.

X. Xantippe

She was born in the Fifth century BC. She was the wife of Socrates. Legend has made her a quarrelsome, shrewish woman.

Y. Loretta Young

She is an American motion picture actress. She won an Academy Award for the film, *The Farmer's Daughter.* (She also appears on television on the late, late show.)

Z. Babe Didrikson Zaharias

She was a great American athlete. She became internationally famous for breaking records. She later devoted herself to golf.

*10.2.9. The Breadfruit Tree**

Introduction (with full voice): Did you know that the breadfruit tree was the cause of a very exciting event in history? You have heard of the mutiny on the *Bounty.* That famous sea saga was the result of this little-known tree.

Part I. A Well-Known Saga

Clue Words

Captain Bligh	specialist	Captain Cook
hero	Caribbean	Tahiti
villain	Brazil	George III
Mutiny on the Bounty	1697	petitioned

Story

Breadfruit was the cause of a well-known saga. It gave Captain Bligh the nickname of Breadfruit Bligh. He was a hero to save the tree. But he was a villain to sailors on the ship *Bounty.* The saga was *The Mutiny on the Bounty.* Bligh was a specialist in shipping valuable plants from one part of the world to another. He shipped breadfruit from the Pacific to the Caribbean. He transferred the rubber tree from Brazil to the Orient. The breadfruit tree was first reported in 1697. Later in the 1770s Captain Cook rediscovered the tree. At the time he was in Tahiti. He sent reports of this tree producing food to King George

*Contributed by Sheila Cornelius, adapted from an article in the *Los Angeles Times,* August 10, 1972.

III of England. Planters petitioned the king to get the trees.

QUESTIONS (use more voice):

1. What was the name of the saga?
2. How was Bligh a hero and a villian?
3. Why was he called a specialist?
4. Why did planters petition King George III?

Part II. A Famous Voyage

Clue Words

devoted	overboard	Jamaica
restless	left	forest
rations	1793	

Story

In 1787 Bligh was sent on his famous voyage. He was devoted to his mission and spent a long time in the South Seas. There he chose 1000 of the best trees he could find. The ship was loaded with these trees, but the men were restless. The situation finally exploded. Bligh had reduced the water rations of the sailors to keep his trees alive. A mutiny followed and the trees were thrown overboard. Bligh was put in a boat and left at sea. He managed to reach land and within a few years returned to get his trees. In 1793 his ship reached Jamaica. It looked like a floating forest. The result was that breadfruit became an important food in the Carribbean.

QUESTIONS:

1. When was Bligh sent on the famous voyage?
2. Why was the situation explosive?
3. What happened to Bligh?
4. When did he reach Jamaica?

Part III. The Breadfruit Tree

Clue Words

fossils	vegetable	cooked
Europe	oval	name
Malaysia	taste	staple

Story

The breadfruit plant is very old. Fossils have been found in Germany. Today the breadfruit cannot be grown anywhere in Europe. It cannot stand frost. It is probably native to Malaysia. This starchy plant became the staple food in the South Pacific. It looks like and is called a fruit, but it is really a vegetable. It is a large, green fruit which is oval in shape. It can weigh up to ten pounds. The taste varies according to when it is picked and how it is cooked. It has been described as tasting like bread, potatoes, and sweet potatoes. Captain Cook said it was completely flavorless. There are over forty edible kinds. The name was invented by Europeans because of its role in tropical diets and because it vaguely resembled fruit.

QUESTIONS:

1. Where were fossils found?
2. Why will breadfruit not grow in Europe?
3. How is it described?
4. Who named it and why?

Part IV. Other Uses of the Breadfruit

Clue Words

milky	boats	leaves
latex	furniture	natives
glue	bark	

Story

For the people in the South Pacific breadfruit has uses other than food. A milky sap comes from the tree when the trunk is cut. This is a latex-like juice. It makes a glue or a kind of vegetable cement. The glue is used for boats and furniture. The bark of the tree is used to make cloth and paper. The large leaves are used as roofing material. The leaves also serve to wrap up food, either for keeping or for cooking.

QUESTIONS:

1. What is made from the milky juice of the tree?
2. What is the glue used for?

3. How is the bark used?
4. How are the leaves used?

Conclude (with voice): Natives prepare the food by cooking the breadfruit in holes in the ground heated with hot stones. Then it is covered with leaves. When the food is soft and charred the skin is scraped off with seashells or coconut shells. It must never be touched with metal (tradition). And now progress! In Hawaii it is prepared and packaged like potato chips— a snack food.

*10.2.10. The Pottery of the Pueblo Indians**

VISUAL AIDS: Pictures of Pueblo Indians and their pottery. Examples of the pottery.

Clue Words

live	hand	shiny
apartment	clay	leaves
cliffs	rubbed	tourists
modern	stone	

EXERCISE SENTENCES:

1. The Pueblo Indians live in the Southwest.
2. They build their homes under cliffs.
3. They make pottery by hand.
4. They make pottery for tourists.
5. It is made today just as it was many years ago.
6. This story tells you how they make their pottery.

Presentation

The Pueblo Indians live in the southwestern part of the United States. They have lived here for many years. Many centuries ago they lived in houses that look like apartment houses. The houses were built under cliffs. This was so they would be protected from the wind and snow. Today the Pueblo Indians live in houses very much the same as ours with all the modern conveniences. The Indians live in the modern world, but they still make their pottery the same way they did many years ago.

*Contributed by Mary Martin and adapted.

Their pottery is all made by hand. First they mix clay and water together. The clay and water are fairly hard. This makes it easier to form into a pot. Once the pot is formed it is rubbed. The Indians rub the outside of the pot smooth with special pieces of stone. When the pot is smooth and shiny it is put into the fire. This makes the pot black. When the pot is finished it comes out shiny. The black pot is then ready to be sold to the tourists.

Recapitulation (teacher points to clue words as she talks): The Pueblo Indians live in the southwestern part of the United States. Their houses looked something like apartments. They were built under cliffs for protection. Today they have modern homes. Their pottery is made by hand. It is made of clay and rubbed hard with a special stone to make it shiny. Wet leaves are put in the fire to make smoke. This turns the pottery black. These shiny black pots are sold to tourists.

10.2.11. London Bridge

Note to the teacher: Do not write the title of the story on the board first, as in most lessons. Ask the students if anyone can lip read without sound, the name of the story you will tell them. Then without voice say, "London Bridge is falling down. . ." If no one is able to answer, give the entire nursery rhyme. Most trained speechreaders will be able to repeat the rhyme with you. Then write the title on the board.

VISUAL AIDS: Pictures of London Bridge and the more familiar Tower Bridge.

Orientation

London Bridge is falling down is a familiar nursery rhyme and children's game. The rhyme is written about the time the first London Bridge came down. Since that time there has been a second London Bridge.

Now there is to be* a third crossing of the Thames at the same place. The history of this famous bridge began centuries ago.

*Note date of completion and alter the sentence.

Part A

Sentences Introduced by Clue Words

Allow for answers and conjectures to the questions.

site	1. Hundreds of years ago there was another bridge at the same place.
Romans	2. Perhaps the first bridge was built by the Romans.
building material	3. What do you think the first bridge was made of?
wood	4. A bridge of wood might fall down after many years.
idea	5. Do you think that is why someone wrote the nursery rhyme?
engineer	6. Many years ago an English bridge builder was called a Bridge Master.
marauders	7. How could a bridge keep out invaders?
church	8. Do you think it would be strange to see a chapel in the middle of a bridge?

Story

About the year 43 AD there was a bridge built at the site of the present London Bridge. No one knows positively who built the bridge. It could have been the Romans. Some believed it was the Britons. There are records that show a bridge has stood on the same site for 1,000 years.

For the next ten centuries the bridges were all made of wood. The last wood bridge is said to have been the inspiration for the nursery rhyme, "London Bridge is falling down. . . " That bridge came down in the year 1014.

Of all the bridges that cross the Thames, none is more famous than London Bridge. There have been two by that name.

Construction on the first London Bridge began in 1176. It was completed thirty-three years later. For 574 years this was the only bridge crossing the Thames. The Bridge Master was Peter de Coelchurch (write).

London Bridge was a masterpiece. It was 905 feet long and twenty feet wide. It was a structure of stone. There were fortified gates to protect the city of London from marauders from the south. Along both sides of the bridge were shops and houses. In the center of the bridge was a chapel.

This bridge lasted for many, many years. The buildings on it gradually wore away and disappeared. Finally it became just a functional bridge serving as a passageway from the south of the city to the north.

Part B

Sentences and Clue Words

eighteenth century	1. The next bridge across the Thames was built about 1750.
destroyed	2. London Bridge, the first, was torn down.
discovery	3. A discovery was made.
foundations	4. What do you think was found at the foundations of the bridge? (try for coins)
proof	5. They found out who built the first bridge.
governing body	6. What do you call the legislature of England? (Parliament)
king	7. When was William IV King of England? (1830-1837)
building materials	8. What do you think was used for building bridges then?
structure	9. What do you think would be used today?

Story

The Thames River had another bridge built across it in 1750. This was Westminster Bridge.

The Old London Bridge was destroyed. Something of historical interest was found on the site of the old structure. Many old Roman coins and medallions were dug up. Because of this fact, it is believed it was the Romans who built a bridge at this same place.

In 1821 Parliament decided to build the second London Bridge. It was opened by William IV in 1831. This was a five-arch bridge of granite. It was 928 feet long and sixty-three feet wide.

Now this second bridge could be said to be "falling down."

The bridge is in no danger. But it is settling very slowly into the river. It is going down at the rate of one-eighth of an inch a year. A tremendous amount of traffic goes over the bridge every day. There is a great need for a larger avenue to take care of the heavy traffic.

The new London Bridge will be made of concrete and steel. It will be a three-span bridge. It will be more streamlined than the former structures. This new bridge will be London Bridge III in good English tradition. It is hoped there will always be a London Bridge.

London Bridge II has been dismantled, stone by stone. It has a new home. The historic span is in the United States. The name remains the same – London Bridge, but add Havasu City, Arizona, U.S.A.

Chapter 11

GAMES AND QUIZZES

A Variety of Contests for Beginning and Advanced Students

A VARIETY OF GAMES and quizzes have been selected for this text. They should provide a change of pace for the intent speechreader of any age. He can now relax and enjoy the fun of participation; for some, games provide a challenge for competing. Many of the games and quizzes are structured not just for entertainment, but to point up basic goals we are trying to reach. This includes increased speechreading skills and the development of a more comprehensive vocabulary. They often increase knowledge in specific areas such as history, geography, and arithmetic.

Any class in speechreading is made up of people with different interests and abilities. For beginning students there are games and quizzes based on everyday language simply stated and more commonplace areas of knowledge. The intermediate and advanced students can read more sophisticated language. This does not imply they are more capable intellectually, but they can usually arrive at answers more rapidly because of speechreading competency. Games or quizzes should be a part of every lesson. They offer variety and fun.

11.1. FOR BEGINNING STUDENTS

*11.1.1. Game to Teach Spacial Relationships**

MATERIALS: Red and blue blocks; blue, yellow, and red cars; a box, a table, and a chair.

PROCEDURE: Two teams, one point given for each correct

*Contributed by Anne Gabriels.

answer. Child must speechread directions and then carry them out.

1. Put the blue block in front of the red block.
2. Put the red block on top of the blue block.

(Repeat the directions using beside, behind, and under)

3. Move the red car forward.
4. Move the blue car backward.
5. Move the yellow car in front of the blue car.

(Continue using between, beside, behind)

Then give directions involving movement in space.

6. John, stand in back of Mary.
7. Jane, stand behind your desk.
8. Mary, stand in front of your desk.

Next, relationship of body to other objects.

9. Jump over a block.
10. Hop around the box.
11. Crawl under the table.
12. Put your hand on the box.
13. Skip to the table and back.
14. Tiptoe around the chair.
15. Walk to the door and back.

*11.1.2. Quiz: House**

PURPOSE: To develop vocabulary related to houses.

Write words on slips of paper and pass out to the class. Whoever has the answer to the question gives the answer.

1. Who builds the house?	carpenter
2. What does the carpenter use to cut the boards?	saw
3. What is used to fasten the boards together?	nails
4. How do you get in the house?	door
5. How do you get up to the house?	sidewalk
6. What makes the house warm?	fireplace
7. What keeps the rain out?	roof
8. What is a room outside the house?	porch
9. What lets the light in?	windows
10. What do you sit on?	chairs

*Contributed by Marion Louks and adapted.

11. What do you walk on?	floor
12. Where do the dishes go?	cupboards
13. How does the smoke come out of the house?	chimney

Note to teacher: Vary the procedure by having flannel board cut-outs of the parts of the house. Let the students place the objects on the board.

11.1.3. Quiz: The Five Senses

PROCEDURE: List the five senses on the board: sight, smell, touch, taste, hearing. The teacher dictates the sentences. Students write only the "sense" indicated by the statement or question. Follow the exercise with questions about each sense as a check on comprehension and recall. For example: Did the clock strike seven or eight?

Student writes—hearing.

Teacher—What did I say about the clock?

taste	1. Chocolate is my favorite kind of ice cream.
sight	2. Our Siamese cat has blue eyes.
touch	3. The fur of a kitten is very soft.
hearing	4. The hum of a mosquito kept me awake last night.
sight	5. I hope I can find a four-leaf clover.
smell	6. What kind of perfume are you wearing?
taste	7. Will you have sugar in your coffee?
hearing	8. Are you afraid of thunder?
smell	9. The air was filled with the odor of pine trees.
touch	10. A blind man's fingers are more sensitive than ours.
hearing	11. He has a very low, bass voice.
sight	12. I love a rainbow!
taste	13. The soup was too salty for me.
touch	14. I burned my hand on the stove.
smell	15. Have you been eating garlic?

11.1.4. Game of Recall on Animal Families, Section 10.1.3.

1. If the baby is called a joey, what is the animal?	kangaroo
2. What strange name is used for a group of geese?	gaggle
3. If the mother bee is a queen, is the father a king?	no, drone

4. Can you name four families of animals in which the mother is called a doe?	deer goat kangaroo rabbit
5. What is the name of a fox father?	Reynard
6. When geese are flying, what is the group called?	skein
7. What would you call the father of a foal?	stallion
8. What is a pride of animals?	lion group
9. What animal lives in a colony?	rabbit
10. Are cats the only animals to have kittens?	no, rabbits

11.1.5. Game of Homophenous Words

Quick Identification for Flexibility and Visual Memory

PROCEDURE: The teacher defines a word. The second word is a homophene for the first word and is some form of plant life, i.e. flower, fruit, shrub, or vegetable.

EXAMPLE:

1. Write a word beginning with M (show manually or place on board) which means the female of a horse.
2. Write the homophenous word which is a fruit.

mare–pear

A. 1. Write a word beginning with R which means arrangements of seats in a theater.
2. Write the homophenous word which is a flower.

rows–rose

B. 1. B_____ another name for seashore.
2. _____ homophene for a fruit.

beach–peach

C. 1. D_____ one-tenth of a dollar.
2. _____ a plant (herb) used for seasoning.

dime–thyme

D. 1. S_____ is a part of a play.
2. _____ the grain of a plant.

scene–seed

E. 1. C_____ a kind of fabric (crinkled).
2. _____ a fruit which grows in clusters.

crepe–grape

F. 1. F____ a struggle, contest, or combat.
2. ____ is a clinging plant.
fight—vine

G. 1. L____ not active.
2. ____ a flower.
lazy—daisy

H. 1. K____ joint of a human found between the thigh and leg.
2. ____ dried leaves of a shrub used to make a drink.
knee—tea

11.1.6. Recognizing the Category

Synonym, Antonym, Homophone, Homophene—Vocabulary Building

PROCEDURE: An explanation of which constitutes each category is given with full voice. The teacher writes the explanation and leaves it on the board for student reference. Examples are placed in this manner.

Synonyms words of same meaning as appetite—craving	*Antonyms* words of opposite meaning as rich—poor
Homophones words that sound alike but have different meaning as colonel—kernel	*Homophenes* words that look alike but are different in meaning as sham—jab

EXAMPLES: The following sentences are given to illustrate the categories. The teacher writes the word vain on the board. Students volunteer to write the paired words found in the following sentences. The students also choose the correct category in which to place the paired words:

1. She is not vain or proud about her appearance. (synonym)
2. She is vain even though her beauty has begun to fade. (homophene)

3. The rooster on the weather vane looks like a vain bird. (homophone)

4. Are you vain or modest about your accomplishments? (antonym)

Sentences

wake	1. Be sure to wake me if I should sleep in class	(antonym)
peace	2. The child gave his mother no peace until she gave him a piece of cake.	(homophone)
which	3. Which would you rather be, beautiful or rich?	(homophene)
sad	4. It made me sad to see the boy so unhappy.	(synonym)
fair	5. When the weather is fair we have a clear view of the ocean.	(synonym)
same	6. They come from the same family but are very different in appearance.	(antonym)
truck	7. A large truck drove up in back of the drugstore.	(homophene)
red	8. She was caught in the rain and her new red dress was soaking wet.	(homophene)
dyed	9. She dyed an old tablecloth a light shade of green.	(homophene)
write	10. The child does not write with his right hand.	(homophone)
planes	11. The planes flew over the plains of the middlewest.	(homophone)
vague	12. He was so vague in giving me directions I was uncertain which way to go.	(synonym)
lost	13. I thought I had lost my key to the house, but I found it in another purse.	(antonym)
knot	14. She tied a knot in her shoe that she could not undo.	(homophone)
last	15. The final game of the season was played on the last day of school.	(synonym)
old	16. If you do not want to become old, spend more time with young people.	(antonym)

11.1.7. A Game with a Message: Why Come to Class?

PROCEDURE: Described by the teacher are words of four letters. Write each word directly below the one above. A student responds after each word described by placing it on the board. It is necessary to have a written response to insure the correct final message. (The message appears vertically in the first and fourth letters.)

1. What word of four letters is the name for a special kind of story? It is a narrative or history of a family. — S A G A
2. Name a small purple fruit often used in a holiday pudding. — P L U M
3. What word of four letters is a very light brown color, the color of unbleached linen? — E C R U
4. What animals are the largest of the deer family? They are also called wapiti. — E L K S
5. What do you call a male horse not more than four years old? — C O L T
6. What is the word for something that is one of two equal parts? — H A L F
7. Can you name a well-known city in western Nevada? Gambling is legal here. — R E N O
8. What word of four letters means always? — E V E R
9. What small island is the farthest west in the Aleutians? — A T T U
10. What name is given to several female animal mothers of fawns, goats, rabbits, antelopes? — D O E S

11.1.8. Games Called Changelings

Changelings appeared in 1879 in the magazine *Vanity Fair.* They were introduced as a game called "Doublets." The author of the game was Charles L. Dodson, better-known as Lewis Carroll, the author of *Alice in Wonderland.**

PROCEDURE: No letter may change position. Only one letter is changed in each successive word. All words in a game have an

---

**The National Observer,* January 1963.

equal number of letters. Each word is written directly below the one above as it is described by the instructor.

Go from Labor to Recreation in Seven Steps

1. What word of four letters means to labor? W O R K
2. Change one letter in work to something you may use when you eat. F O R K
3. Change one letter in fork to a word meaning shape or frame. F O R M
4. Change a letter in form to something you may see on a wave at the beach. F O A M
5. What word of four letters means nonsense, humbug, or a falsehood? F L A M
6. What word of four letters means to strip off skin or to criticize severely? F L A Y
7. Change a letter in flay to have a word that means recreation. P L A Y

*11.1.9. What We Want to See at Ball Games—six steps**

1. What four-letter word is where most of us will go after class? H O M E
2. Change home into a word meaning a way to sharpen a razor. H O N E
3. Change one letter in hone to a word meaning finished, like a good job. D O N E
4. What is a word of four letters meaning Spanish gentlemen—a title of courtesy? D O N S
5. Change dons to a word meaning a demand for money —ask for payment. D U N S
6. What word means goes fast on foot in a ball game? R U N S

11.1.10. Make Home Out of Barn in Six Steps

1. What word of four letters is a building found on a farm to house animals? B A R N
2. Change one letter in barn to have a word meaning stripped naked. B A R E

*Contributed by Cora Sydnor.

3. Change a letter in bare to make a word for a small animal with long ears. — H A R E
4. What word of four letters will change hare to a word meaning healthy or vigorous? — H A L E
5. Change one letter in hale for a word which means an excavation or a pit. — H O L E
6. By changing one letter in hole can you make a word for a dwelling—a place to live? — H O M E

11.1.11. Make something Good to Eat in Nine Steps

1. What word of five letters is a grain that is ground to make flour for baking? — W H E A T
2. Change a letter in wheat to form the word meaning to swindle or deceive. — C H E A T
3. Can you change cheat to a five-letter word meaning marked down in price? — C H E A P
4. Change cheap to a word of five letters meaning a sound made by a bird. — C H E E P
5. Change a letter in cheep to a word that describes the way a baby moves along. — C R E E P
6. What word of five letters changes creep to a word meaning faith or belief? — C R E E D
7. Change a letter in creed for a word meaning an extreme desire for something. — G R E E D
8. Can you change one letter in greed to make a word meaning family or pedigree? — B R E E D
9. What word of five letters is a food made out of wheat flour? — B R E A D

11.2. INTERMEDIATE LEVEL

11.2.1. Arbor Day Game

A brief description of each tree is given for clues. The students fill in the blank spaces indicated by the dashes.

PROCEDURES: Draw the tree outline on the board. Put in the letters and dashes. The students draw the same tree on paper. Explain the dashes represent the proper number of letters in each

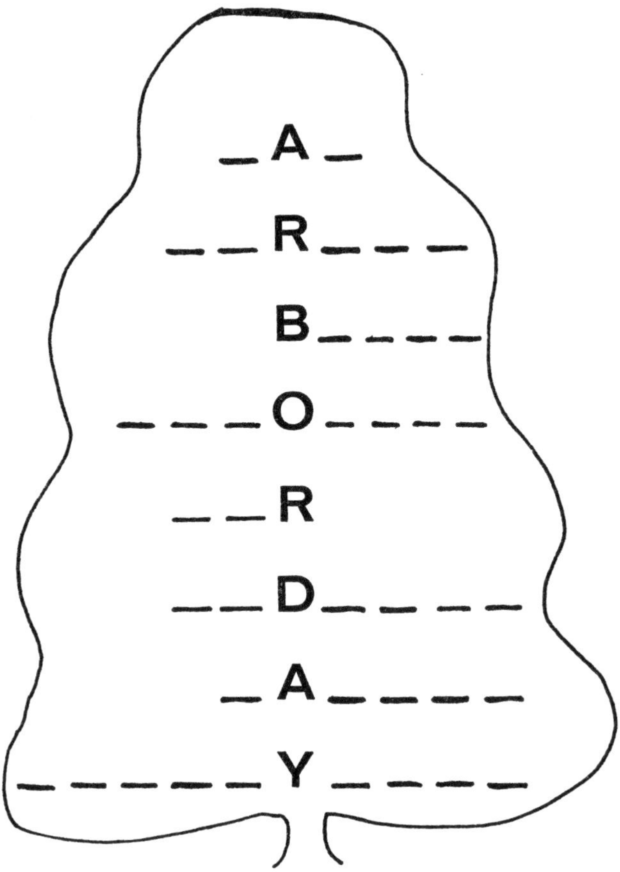

Figure 33.

tree to be described. At the end of the exercise volunteers take turns filling in the spaces one line at a time. Each volunteer gives the substance of the description read by the teacher. The clue words are written on the board after the tree has been drawn. Clue words may not be necessary for upper grade levels. This provides the students with an opportunity to anticipate the language. Go over the words with and without voice.

Clue Words

acorns	furniture	nuts
evergreen	Christmas	Australia
bark	Pacific coast	

1. This is a large tree. It has spreading branches. The wood of this tree is tough and hard. The tree produces acorns. — O A K
2. This tree is an evergreen. It is a handsome tree with heavy foliage or needles. It is a tall tree with bluish-green foliage. — S P R U C E
3. The bark of this tree is used for many things. American Indians used the bark of this tree to cover their boats. The boats were called canoes. — B I R C H
4. The wood of this tree is very valuable. It is used to make fine furniture. — M A H O G A N Y
5. This tree is often used at Christmas time. It is a pine tree. Some of these trees are very fragrant. — F I R
6. This tree grows in California (Pacific Coast). It grows very tall. Some of these trees live for hundreds of years. — R E D W O O D
7. This tree is a beautiful shade tree. The wood is valuable for furniture. The fruit or nuts are an important food. — W A L N U T
8. This is an Australian tree. It is the home of the Koala bear. The oil from the tree is used in medicine. — E U C A L Y P T U S

11.2.2. A New Word for Speechreading

Procedure: The teacher says, "When this game is completed you will have a familiar term and a medical word both meaning speechreading." Number from one to ten horizontally. The described words are all three-letter words. All words are written vertically under the numbers. The answers to the words may be written on the board by volunteers, or each may write at his desk.

1. Start with L, end with L —have a girl's nickname (LIL)
2. Start with I, end with A —letters represent International Phonetic Alphabet (IPA)
3. Start with P, end with B —the name for an English tavern (PUB)
4. Start with R, end with I —French word for king (ROI)
5. Start with E, end with O—means the complete person (EGO)
6. Start with A, end with M—a limb of your body, shoulder, wrist (ARM)
7. Start with D, end with A —three letters used to name a body chemical (DNA)
8. Start with I, end with N—a place for food and lodging (INN)
9. Start with N, end with C —familiar TV channel (NBC)
10. Start with G, end with Y —means joyous, happy; a slang word with a different connotation (GAY)

Labiomancy is medically defined for lipreading; from Latin *labium* meaning lip and Greek *manteia* meaning divination.

*11.2.3. A Word Game—Synonyms We Should Know**

Procedure: A word is written on the board. The teacher then gives several sentences containing synonyms for the first written word. The teacher says, "See if you can identify them."

1. Adequate
   The stenographer was a *capable* worker.
   That is the end of the meal; have you had *sufficient?*
   The tired runner had jogged *enough.*
   The average student made *satisfactory* grades.

2. Affluent
   Money makes a man *rich.*
   The *wealthy* family lived in a mansion.
   The jet-set are among the *well-to-do.*

*Contributed by Judith Porter.

3. Defects
   The earthquake occurred on the *fault.*
   Some people try to hide their *weaknesses.*
   The *flaw* was barely visible in her diamond.
   Hand-made sweaters often show *imperfections.*
4. Genuine
   The stone was a *true* sapphire.
   Where is the *correct* Howard Hughes will?
   Better stores maintain an *honesty* in merchandise.
5. Appropriate
   Well-mannered people take the *proper* action.
   The woman searched for the *right* man.
   Suitable flowers glorify any occasion.
6. Donate
   Will you *furnish* your silver coffee service for the party?
   The man offered to *supply* his talents.
   Give to your favorite charity.
   We are here to *present* you with a scholarship.
7. Charter
   The sign read, "Apartment for *lease.*"
   The wealthy woman *hired* a private plane.
   He *employs* a Certified Public Accountant.
8. Concise
   Short paragraphs are still informative.
   The lawyer prepared a *brief.*
   The teacher enjoyed *pithy* answers.
9. Illiterate
   The *ignorant* cannot read or write.
   The *unlearned* are not always those who missed school.
   She *lacks* knowledge in the field of music.
10. Hazardous
   The winding trail was *dangerous.*
   Rain made the road a *risk* to travel.
   The soldier had *perilous* duty on the front lines.

11.2.4. Plants with Animal Names—A Game or Contest

PROCEDURE: The blank spaces are filled in with the names of animals. The completed words are the names of well-known plants. Each blank represents a letter.

Example: _ _ _ _ stool (toadstool)
Add a jumping amphibian and you will have a mushroom.

1. _ _ _ _ grass (crabgrass)
Add a crustacean and the plant is a strong grass that invades lawns.
2. _ _ _ wood (dogwood)
Add an animal called man's best friend, and you have a plant or tree that is the state flower of Virginia and North Carolina.
3. _ _ _ _ _ cabbage (skunkcabbage)
Add a small animal capable of giving off a very strong odor and the plant is a small herb also capable of having a strong odor.
4. _ _ _ tail (cattail)
Add an animal kept as a pet (it purrs when it is happy), and you have a tall marsh plant with a long cylinder of brown flowers.
5. _ _ _ _ eye (buckeye)
Add the male of the deer family and the plant is a native shrub or tree of Ohio.
6. _ _ _ _ bell (harebell)
Add a rabbit and you have a flower that is sometimes called a bluebell.
7. _ _ _ _ grass (beargrass)
Add a large, powerful wild animal found in western North America, and the plant is a species of yucca (lily).
8. _ _ _ _ _ willow (pussywillow)
Add a pet name for a cat, and the plant will be a flower-like cluster on willow trees.
9. _ _ _ _ _ berry (gooseberry)
Add a bird with a long neck, related to the swan, and you have a shrub producing berries fit for a pie.

11.3. ADVANCED LEVEL

*11.3.1. European Geography—A Quiz**

PROCEDURE: The information about these places can be used

*Contributed by Lola Mendez.

as a quiz or as a participation exercise. If it is used as a quiz the students may write the answers. When the quiz is finished volunteers may offer to give as much information as they can remember about one place or thing. If used as a participation exercise, slips may be prepared for each place to be described. The students work together in pairs or in groups of three or four. Each student takes a turn reading all of the information on his slip.

Clue Words (on Board)

town	lake	river	capital
hill	church	island	colony
city	bell	country	sea
building			

Go over the words with and without voice until all are recognized. It is necessary for each student to read the categories because this important clue is given in the first sentence.

1. This is a sea. It is one of the most treacherous seas in the world. It is often rough, stormy, and covered by fog. This sea produces more fish than any other body of water in the world. It is between Scandinavia and Great Britain. What sea is it? *The North Sea*

2. This is a famous river. It flows between two countries. There are beautiful old castles on the banks of this river. Boats take sightseers along this river. It flows between France and Germany. What river is it? *The Rhine*

3. This is a building. It is a huge structure nearly 1,000 feet high. It was built for the World's Exposition in 1889. It was designed by the same man who designed the framework for the Statue of Liberty. It is in Paris, France. What structure is it? *The Eiffel Tower*

4. This is a country. It has a reputation for being very clean. The people work hard to keep out the North Sea. It is famous for cheese. It exports tons of tulip bulbs every year. This country is ruled by a queen. What is the name of the country? *The Netherlands*

5. This is an island. It is the largest island in the world. Four-fifths of this island lies under an icecap. The people who live here are Eskimos. The population is about 25,000. The island is a part of the Danish kingdom. What island is it? *Greenland*

6. This is a capital. It is about sixty miles from the North Sea. This city is famous for its charm and beauty. It is a fashion and art center. It is famous for the manufacture of lace. Some of the most beautiful tapestries in the world are made here. What capital is it? *Brussels*

7. This is a country. It is a large island. The northern part of this country has industries. The southern part has farms. The northern part is also a part of the British Commonwealth. The southern part is independent. Can you name the country? *Ireland*

8. This is a hill. It is the highest hill in the city. There is the ruin of a famous temple here. The city is Athens, Greece. The ruin is the Parthenon. What is the name of the hill? *Acropolis*

9. This is a town. It is in England, not far from London. There is an observatory here. A meridian passes through this town. When the sun crosses that meridian, standard time begins. What town is this? *Greenwich*

10. This is a large church. It stands on an island in the Seine River. The architecture of the church is Gothic. It has flying buttresses. It is in Paris, France. What is the name of this cathedral? *Notre Dame*

11. This was a small city. It was a beautiful summer resort in ancient Roman days. The city was destroyed when Vesuvius erupted. The city was covered with ashes. This happened in the year 79 AD. Excavations have shown what life in ancient Italy was like. What city is it? *Pompeii*

12. This is a lake. It is the largest inland body of water in the world. It is a salt lake. It is 92 feet below sea level. Four-fifths of its shoreline is in Russia. It covers an area of 163,800

square miles. What lake is it? (may add: The lake is called a sea.) *Caspian Sea*

13. This is a huge bell. It is in a clock tower in London, England. The tower is at the north end of the Parliament Building. The bell weighs 13½ tons and was cast in 1858. The name of the bell is usually given to the clock in the tower. What bell is it? *Big Ben*

14. This is a group of stone buildings. They were built as a castle. They are in London, England. At one time they were used as a prison. Many famous people were put to death here. The Crown Jewels are guarded here. By what name is it known? *The Tower of London*

15. This is a colony. It is a Crown Colony southeast of Spain. It guards the entrance to the Mediterranean. There is a huge rock here, 1,396 feet high. At the foot of the rock is an important naval base. What colony is it? *Gibraltar*

*11.3.2. Getting To Know You**

PROCEDURE: Divide the class into groups of two. Give one partner in each group a card with the directions for each stage of talk. Alternate the card placement.

Introduction (given in full voice to the entire class): Talking is one way of knowing others. Talking can also be a way of keeping others from knowing us. This game can help show you how talk can let others know you or keep others from knowing you. Think of yourself as having a large circle around you. Some people we keep out to the farthest perimeter. Other people we let in a little closer. A few people we let in to the center of our circle. Let's play a game so that you can get the feel of what I am saying.

Arms Length Talk

(full voice) I call this first part "Arms Length Talk." One partner will use reduced voice and repeat one of the following sentences to the other partner. The receiving partner will re-

*This game is adapted from the book, *Why Am I Afraid to Tell You Who I Am?* by Powell. Contributed by Judith Porter.

spond in full voice. When you finish the following sentences, feel free to add some of your own.

Card I (reduced voice)

How are you?
How is your family?
Where have you been?
I hope we can get together real soon.
I'm fine.
What have you been doing?
What's new?
How do you like the weather?
Good to see you.
Sorry to hear that.
It looks like rain.
Happy to meet you.
That's too bad.
Hope we meet again.
What do you know?
How are you feeling?

Fending Off Talk

(full voice) The second stage I call "Fending Off Talk." At this level you will only be able to report facts and stories about others. In reduced voice one partner will start the sentences on the card (printed below) and then finish them in his own words. The other partner will respond in full voice. When finished, alternate the card and let the second partner finish his own sentences.

Card II (reduced voice)

My friend told me that . . .
My sister (brother) is . . .
Last week my neighbor . . .
The newspaper said that . . .
The weather is . . .
The waitress told me . . .
The instructor said . . .

Let me tell you what ______ said . . .
Let me tell you what ______ did . . .
Let me tell you what ______ said about . . .

I Think Talk

(full voice) This stage I call "I think talk." The speaker tells you about his thoughts and judgments. This is the first time the speaker has told you anything about himself. As a listener and responder it is important to accept the thoughts and judgments as given. If the speaker observes even one raised eyebrow, he might stop talking. He might stop telling about himself and begin saying what he thinks the listener wants to hear.

Use the same format as last time. Finish the statements with your own answer. Omit those that do not apply to you. Feel free to make up your own.

Card III (reduced voice)

I think taxes are . . .
I think we should change . . .
______ should wear a different . . .
My daughter's (son's) wedding was . . .
The movies these days are . . .
All large dogs are . . .
I think you should . . .
I think he (she) should . . .
I think they are . . .
I think the world is . . .
Children these days are . . .
I think hearing aids are . . .
The President should . . .
I believe in . . .
I plan to vote for . . .

I Feel Talk

(full voice) The last stage I call "I feel talk." The speaker allows the listener to be in the center of his circle: "I want to tell you about my feelings; if I trust you, I may tell you about my feelings at this moment." You may find it difficult to talk only about your feelings. We seem to be more relaxed when talking about our thoughts.

Follow the same format. Finish each statement with your own feelings.

Card IV (reduced voice)

I like the way you . . .
I am . . .
I feel . . . in this group.
At this moment I . . .
My stomach is . . .
My throat is . . .

The instructor may like to encourage a group discussion following the completion of the game.

Chapter 12

CONVERSATIONS AND SKITS

For Two or Three Speakers

CONVERSATIONS AND SKITS may be successfully used for all levels of speechreaders. Prepared materials vary in complexity depending on the ability level of the participants.

For beginning speechreaders the skit or conversation should have colloquial language based on familiar topics. The conversation is prepared and scripts are given long enough ahead of time for the students to practice. The "actors" should be familiar with the script so they can simulate a natural conversational situation. When two are giving the skit they should face each other and the class at a slight angle so all may observe expressions and hear the dialogue. The rate of speech must be slightly slower than ordinary conversation to allow the "audience" to follow the story while watching the exchange of talk.

At the intermediate or advanced level a skit may include three or more speakers. A skit of this kind requires the spectators and participants to watch closely as the conversation crosses from one speaker to another. It is tiring and more difficult, and for this reason should be limited to brief periods of time.

Conversations and skits may be given by two or more participants in front of the class, or there may be several skits going on at one time. Another way of presentation is for the pupils to sit in a circle and talk with a person directly across from him. It is necessary for all to use full voice. This means they will be subjected to ambient talk and laughter interfering with concentration and the ability to block out these extraneous sounds. This speechreading exercise is good practice, for it creates the kind of situation the hard-of-hearing individual has to face in groups or at a party.

12.1. PLAYING CATCH

Script for Participant A (Talkers speak in turn)

1. Let's play catch after school tonight.
2. Your place. Your mother feeds us.
3. I'll be there around four o'clock. I have to go home first.
4. Oh, Boy. I can taste that chocolate cake right now.
5. Maybe we should play at my house then.

Script for Participant B

1. O.K. Shall we play at school or at my place?
2. O.K. When can you come?
3. All right. I'll tell my mother you're coming. Maybe she'll get the hint.
4. Sorry. I finished the last piece of it last night.
5. What's your mother got to eat?

12.2 CHRISTMAS GIFTS

1\. Did you have a nice Christmas?
2\. Oh, yes, it was exciting at our house.
1\. At ours too. What happened at your house?
2\. My dad was Santa Claus for my little brother. He came to the door and brought a train for Bobby.
1\. I wish I could have seen him. Did *that* Santa Claus bring you anything?
2\. *That* Santa Claus brought me everything I wanted.
1\. I was lucky too. I got a radio and boots.
2\. Do you want to know the most exciting thing of all?
1\. Tell me what was so exciting.
2\. I'm going to have my own telephone in my room.
1\. Call me the minute you get it.
2\. I'll do that.

12.3. JIMMY AND HIS MOTHER ON THE WAY TO THE MOVIES*

Introduce (with full voice): Jimmy and his mother have been shopping. They have left the store and are walking up the street.

Jimmy: Where are we going now, Mom?
Mother: How would you like to go to a movie, Jimmy?
J: Great! I wanna see a western.
M: Well, this is a good show, but it isn't a western.
J: Gee, I don't wanna see any ol' love story.
M: This isn't a love story. But you'll like it; just wait and see.
J: What's it about? What's it called?
M: It's *The Big Top*. (more voice)
J: What's that? That doesn't sound so wonderful.
M: Maybe you'll be surprised. You like clowns, don't you?
J: Sure. They're O.K.
M: How about wild animals and horses that do tricks?
J: You mean like elephants and tigers? Is it a circus?
M: Yes, that's what *Big Top* means—circus.
J: (taking his mother's hand and pulling her along) Come on—let's hurry. Can I have some popcorn and soda pop?
M: For goodness sake! All you ever think about is eating!
J: Gee, Mom, a guy's gotta eat.
M: Well, I suppose so. (Aside) What's a circus without popcorn—Maybe I'll have some myself.

12.4. BASEBALL – CROSS CONVERSATION FOR THREE*

A. 1. Are you going out for the baseball team this year?
   2. I don't care, just so I make the team.
   3. He plays for the *Giants*.
   4. The parade was called off because it rained.

B. 1. I sure am. I hope I'll make it this time. Are you?
   2. Then maybe you can play centerfield like Mickey Mantle.

---

*Contributed by Ruth Reed and adapted.

*Cross conversation with rapid topic change is a more difficult advanced exercise.

3. I saw a giant at the circus last night.
4. Just like baseball.

C. 1. Yes, I am. But this year I want to play shortstop. What do you want to play?
2. I'd like to steal bases like Lou Brock.
3. Did you see the parade?
4. Let's practice so we can make the team.

12.5. WHAT DID YOU THINK OF THAT TEST – TOPIC CHANGE†

Fred: What did you think of that test?
Sam: Absolutely awful!
Fred: Man, he didn't ask one thing on the material I studied.
Sam: Well, I knew the material, but I just couldn't get it down on paper; you know how it is during this spring weather.
Fred: Yeah, I don't know how he expects this stuff about biology to help me, a business major. I'd rather be fishing.
Sam: Me, too, but I have to get a "B" in this class or I can't graduate this June.
Fred: No kiddin'.
Sam: I don't know why he gives so much outside work when I have other stuff to do.
Fred: Well, I'm not going to worry about it. I've got to get home to clean up for the party tonight–you coming?
Sam: I don't know. Last night was too much for me. I didn't get home until three–who's going?
Fred: I heard those cute girls in biology class talking about it.
Sam: On second thought–I'll be there.

12.6. BUYING SHOES – A CUSTOMER AND SALESMAN*

S: Good afternoon. May I help you?
C: Yes. I'd like to see some shoes for fall–something in brown.
S: Of course. What size do you wear?
C: 7-B.
S: (Bringing out several pairs of shoes) How do you like these?

---

†Contributed by Deril Schmitt and adapted.
*Contributed by Kay Schneider and adapted.

C: (Selecting a pair, saying) Let me try these—Ouch! These are too tight!
S: Perhaps you should take a $7\frac{1}{2}$. Let me check your shoe size.
C: No, I take a 7-B. Your shoes could be marked wrong.
S: How about these?
C: I think the heel is too high.
S: Maybe you would like this pair?
C: Oh. They look so square!
S: Madam, this is a very smart new style.
C: They look square to me.
S: Try this pair on.
C: Very comfortable—nice heel—How much are they?
S: A bargain today—only sixteen dollars.
C: Perfect. I'll take them.
S: Shall I wrap them or will you wear them?
C: I'll wear them. They're so comfortable.
S: (speaks in an aside as she leaves) They're $7\frac{1}{2}$s!

12.7. AFTER HIGH SCHOOL, WHAT NEXT? – TOPIC CHANGES

A. Have you made up your mind what you are going to do when you finish school?
B. Not for sure. But my folks want me to go to college. What about you?
A. I think I would like to go to a vocational school.
B. What would you study?
A. Mechanics. I have already taken my car apart twice. I know every part and where it belongs.
B. I wish I did. When something goes wrong with mine it costs me plenty.
A. Where do you think you will go to school?
B. I'll probably go to a Junior College. What I'd really like to do is travel a year.
A. I would, too, but I don't have the money.
B. Neither do I, but I'm going to try to find something where I can earn as I go.
A. I may have a chance to drive some relatives across the country.

B. Sounds great. I'd like to get some job—any job—on a steamship line for the summer.

A. Well, good luck.

B. Same to you.

12.8. IN LINE AT THE CAFETERIA – SKIT FOR THREE*

A. I wonder what they're having in the cafeteria today.

B. I hope it's good.

C. Me too. I'm starving. I didn't eat breakfast this morning.

A. You should, you know.

C. I know, but I didn't have time. I had an eight o'clock class this morning.

B. Is that your speech class? How's your teacher?

C. He's pretty good. I had him for another class last year.

A. So did I. He was great.

B. Why isn't this line moving any faster?

C. There are only two people working.

A. Why don't they hire more people?

B. You'd think they could afford it.

C. I know, with all the money they're saving on the food they give us here.

A. Can you see what they're serving?

B. Spaghetti or beef dip.

C. Oh, good. That's not bad and I'm starving.

A. I just had spaghetti last night.

B. Oh, that reminds me—did you try that new recipe?

C. Do you mean the one I gave you last week?

A. I'm going to try it tomorrow night. There's a special on at the market.

B. Oh, yes, I saw that in the paper today.

C. Here we are finally. Gosh, I'm starving.

A. I'll have spaghetti.

B. Beef dip, please.

C. Could I have the beef dip open-faced?

A. I'll get the drinks.

B. Where shall we sit?

---

*Contributed by Linda Yamasaki.

C. How about that seat by the window?
A. My spaghetti is cold!
B. The beef dip is lousy!
C. I'm starving!

12.9. WHAT WIVES SAY IN THE MORNING*

A one-way conversation, wife to husband. This should be dramatized for the best effect. The husband pantomimes his responses after each sentence given by the wife.

1. It's time to get up.
2. Here is your clean shirt.
3. The coffee is ready.
4. Your tie is crooked.
5. Did you get a clean handkerchief?
6. Would you like some orange juice?
7. The milkman hasn't come yet so you'll have to drink your coffee black.
8. Are your eggs cooked enough?
9. I'll start the car.
10. You forgot your briefcase.
11. What time will you be home?
12. Dinner will be ready at six sharp.
13. I hope you will not be late for work.
14. You will have to hurry.
15. Have a good day at the office.
16. Oh! Oh! I forgot to put gas in the car yesterday.
17. Sorry dear!

---

*Contributed by Alta Taylor and adapted.

Chapter 13

THE GOSPEL ACCORDING TO SPEECHREADING

The Do's and Don'ts for the Hearing-Impaired

SPEECHREADING IS THE GROSS PROCESS of looking at, listening to, perceiving, and interpreting spoken symbols. But since many of the symbols are not visible or audible, a good deal of "educated guessing" is often necessary in order to understand what has been said.

Give Yourself a Break

1. Be kind to yourself. It is not your fault that you have a hearing loss, so don't blame yourself for it and don't apologize to others.
2. Stand far enough back to see the speaker's face.
3. Be willing to ask people to repeat.
4. Be sure that the other person is not embarrassed by your inability to hear; don't bluff. It is stupid and rude.
5. Keep sociable. Cultivate your friends. Tell your friends you have a problem; most want to help.
6. When you enter a room "Case the joint"; be sure you are not interrupting a conversation in progress.
7. Avoid saying *what* before the speaker has completed a sentence. You may get the meaning if you wait.
8. Have a wide variety of interests and keep abreast of what is going on in the world so you can contribute.

---

*Adapted and modified, source unknown.

There Are Multiple Cues That Help Us to Understand Speech

1. *Listening.* Try not to take over. Many hard of hearing dominate the conversation. If you are talking you don't know what has been said!
2. *Watching the Speaker.* It takes time to catch on and follow unfamiliar speech patterns.
3. *Feeling Movement.* You can tell by feeling the vibrations on your throat and face if you are speaking too loudly or too softly. You can also sometimes guess what the speaker is saying if you imitate his movements, but don't be obvious about it.
4. *Interpreting Situational Clues.* For example:
   a. *Facial Expression.* Emotion is usually shown on the face of the speaker. Few people are dead pan when angry or happy. An angry person looks angry. This may provide a clue to what he is about to say.
   b. *Body Language.* Gestures, movements of the head, hands, arms, feet, or entire body tell a lot. Example–a fanning or mopping motion often accompanies conversation about hot weather.
   c. *Objects.* The presence of any object on which the speaker is focusing may provide a clue to what he may say. Example–A pencil with a broken point suggests that something may be said about sharpening the pencil or obtaining another.
   d. *Person Talking.* Frequently it is possible to anticipate and to know almost exactly what a person is going to say as soon as that person is seen.
   e. *Place Conversation is Held.* In many situations the conversation follows a usual pattern. Example–In a restaurant the conversation with the waiter would be very different from the conversation in a doctor's office.

Aids to Good Speechreading

1. Relax. Don't try so hard you become tense and frustrated. Roll with the punches.
2. Be alert.

3. Be confident.
4. Be determined to understand.
5. Follow every clue. Improve your powers of observation. Everyone can do it. Make the most of your residual hearing.
6. Be interested in what is going on.
7. Do not try to follow every word people say. The key words which unlock the meaning may be at the end of the sentence. Therefore, you must let your eyes travel over the words until the speaker pauses.
8. Practice whenever possible: eavesdrop and eyedrop! Example—If you go to a restaurant for food, try to read the waitress and the other customers.

Suggestions for Someone Who Might Help You at Home

1. Always have the light on the speaker's face. (What do you do? Maneuver without being obvious.)
2. Speak clearly and naturally, but beware of exaggeration and mouthing, that is, moving the lips and jaw in an unnatural manner.
3. Speak with voice; *never give silent instruction.* It is unnatural.
4. Know the material well enough to be able to keep your head up so that the student can see the complete action of the lips and tongue and can have the advantage of facial expression and clear audition.
5. Avoid unnatural movement of the hands. This can be very distracting.
6. Do not give an undue amount of repetition. If the student does not understand after the second time, change the words but retain the context. If necessary give one of the important words with more voice. Example—It's a nice day. Change to: This is a beautiful day.
7. Rarely repeat single words. It's usually better to repeat the entire idea.
8. Three fifteen-minute practice periods a day are preferable, but a maximum of forty-five minutes at one sitting is satisfactory. Don't overdo it. Fatigue may result in discouragement. Some days are better than others.

Suggestions for the Speechreader

1. *Practice your speechreading at all times.* Having developed basic skill in a classroom situation, practice on the outside. Many everyday experiences offer opportunity for practice. Look while you listen.
2. *Give undivided, relaxed attention to the speaker.* He may be laboring to slow down his usual rapid speaking pace and he may be exerting the utmost patience, all for your benefit. Therefore, you should do him the kindness of concentrating on his speech to the best of your ability. The burden is on you. So use a little flattery. Let him know you are interested in what he is saying and ask questions about what you missed.
3. *Develop mental alertness.* The more you practice using your powers of imagination and anticipation, the better your speechreading will be.
4. *Use your imagination.* If you get only one or two words you can often decide what the other words are, or at least get the meaning, if you stop and think about it. Lip formation, mouth opening, facial expression, expectation, imagination, and intuition all figure in speech interpretation.
5. *Remember.* Lipreading is more correctly termed Speechreading. Do not make hard work of it by concentrating entirely on lip formations. A person's entire countenance is expressive of what he is saying.
6. *Read current literature.* Lack of familiarity with some expression a person may be using only adds to the difficulty of speechreading, so keep your vocabulary up-to-date by reading as many newspapers, magazines, and books as possible. Know what people are talking about.
7. *Get enough rest.* At all times there is a certain amount of nervous strain on the speechreader; since you cannot concentrate as well when tired and nervous, an extra amount of relaxation is necessary in order to be alert when spoken to.
8. *Do not be discouraged.* Learning speechreading takes time and practice. Even some of the experts have blank spells when they cannot read speech any better than a novice does. You are not the only one who has an occasional mental block.

The 3 Ps (paraphrased from the 3 Rs): Patience, Practice, and Perseverance. You may gain expertise with the speed of a glacier. How long will it take? The rest of your life!

9. *Never indulge in self-pity.* This is easy to do but will not win friends and influence people. The hearing person usually tries to help. The hard-of-hearing person has a twenty-four-hour problem that is comparable to a bad telephone connection: strain—exhausted after a few minutes.
10. *Keep your sense of humor active.* To be able to laugh at your own misinterpretations makes it easier for yourself as well as for others, and the better natured you are, the more people will want to talk to you. Don't ever act annoyed, even though you are annoyed with yourself.
11. *People are different.* Remember learning this skill is not an easy job accomplished in ten lessons. It takes time. Never compare your ability to that of your neighbor. Compare yourself with yourself. There is no criterion except to improve your own ability. Remember what Benjamin Franklin said, circa 1750: "When you speak to a man look in his eyes. When he speaks to you, look in his mouth."

Appendix

JEFFER'S SPEECH AND SOUND RECOGNITION TEST*

Introduction

THE JEFFER'S SPEECH SOUND RECOGNITION TEST (SSRT) is a test of a person's ability to recognize individual speech sounds. It is useful in obtaining an indication of the speechreading ability for the child whose insufficient language prohibits the use of other standard speechreading instruments. The SSRT has also proved to be useful with non-English speaking adults or children (or those who have limited command of the English language).

Test Description

There are two parts to the test—actually two tests—one for the perception of the vowel sounds and one for the perception of consonant sounds. The sounds are listed in the first column. The two adjacent columns provide for the examiner's recording of the (correct/incorrect) response under two test conditions—look and listen, and listen.

Administration

The test should be given in a quiet, well-lighted room with a minimum of distractions. The examiner should be seated approximately three feet in front of (and facing) the examinee. The examiner indicates to the examinee that he is to imitate the sounds about to be made. (This can usually be accomplished through gestures.) The examiner then presents the sounds as listed in Table II, using a normal voice level. Consonant sounds are

*Edited by Shirley Oakes.

TABLE II

Sound In Isolation	1. Speechreading (Look and Listen)	2. Hearing (Listen Only)
	mouth in full	mouth
	view	covered
b		
d		
g		
z		
y		
ð (th)		
dʒ		
ʒ (zh)		
m		
n		
ŋ (ng)		
l		
r		
w		
hw		
j (you)		
p		
t		
k		
s		
ʃ (sh)		
tʃ (ch)		
f		
θ		
h		
i (tree)		
ɪ (pig)		
eɪ (cake)		
ɛ (bed)		
æ (cat)		
ɝ (bird)		
ʌ (cup)		
u (shoe)		
ʊ (book)		
oʊ (boat)		
ɔ (ball)		
ɑ (sock)		
ɑɪ (pie)		
ɑʊ (cow)		
ɔɪ (boy)		

1. Consonants ____/25____% 2. Consonants ____/25____%

Vowels ____/15____% Vowels ____/15____%

TOTAL ____/40____% TOTAL ____/40____%

given either in isolation or followed by the schwa. Vowel sounds are given in isolation or in a simple word, e.g. *tree,* to elicit the /i/ sound.

The list of sounds is presented twice, first with the examiner's mouth in full view, and then with the examiner's mouth being completely covered (an 8 by 11 piece of cardboard is recommended—a thin paper sometimes moves in response to plosive air streams). Make a blue check if sound is correct; make a red X if missed. Record sound substitutions, e.g. p/b (p for b).

Scoring and Interpretation

If a person receives a score of 50 percent on the "listen" portion of the test, and 100 percent on the "look and listen" portion, it is apparent that this person is using his vision (at least for isolation speech sounds) to aid in communication. If, however, his scores are 50 percent and 50 percent, his vision is not contributing to information received. In addition to this general interpretation, specific speech sound discrimination difficulties can be analyzed, providing a base for both auditory and visual remediation programs.

INDEX

T

V

Y